Bad Foods

Bad Foods

Changing Attitudes About What We Eat

Michael E. Oakes

Transaction Publishers
New Brunswick (U.S.A.) and London (U.K.)

Copyright © 2004 by Transaction Publishers, New Brunswick, New Jersey.

All rights reserved under International and Pan-American Copyright Conventions. No part of this book may be reproduced or transmitted in any form or by any means, electronic or mechanical, including photocopy, recording, or any information storage and retrieval system, without prior permission in writing from the publisher. All inquiries should be addressed to Transaction Publishers, Rutgers—The State University, 35 Berrue Circle, Piscataway, New Jersey 08854-8042.

This book is printed on acid-free paper that meets the American National Standard for Permanence of Paper for Printed Library Materials.

Library of Congress Catalog Number: 2004046057
ISBN: 0-7658-0228-7
Printed in Canada

Library of Congress Cataloging-in-Publication Data

Oakes, Michael E.
    Bad foods : changing attitudes about what we eat / Michael E. Oakes.
        p. cm.
    Includes bibliographical references and index.
    ISBN 0-7658-0228-7 (alk. paper)
        1. Nutrition—United States—Public opinion. 2. Food habits—United States. I. Title.

QP141.O24   2004
613.2'0973—dc22   2004046057

Contents

Acknowledgments

I was born with a rare visual impairment. The completion of this volume, which took a matter of months, would have otherwise required years had it not been for the help of my wife and research partner (Carole Slotterback) who did the bulk of the library work while I focused on writing *Bad Foods*. I will always be in gratitude to her, whenever things appeared bleak Carole stood tall, her encouragement was unwavering.

Also, I want to thank the dozens of University of Scranton students who both assisted and motivated me in my research endeavors. The students who were particularly inspiring in getting this research off the ground and, thus, deserve special thanks are Steve Lukasik, Christy Piedmont, and Pam Palumbo.

Additionally, I am most grateful to the librarians at the University of Scranton who acquired the hundreds of references for this book without complaint (at least none that I could hear).

Finally, I am thankful to the journal editors and reviewers who over the years welcomed this unorthodox and controversial inquiry.

1

What's in a Name?

Those of us who live in the United States are inclined more than people from any other developed country in the world to have food-related problems. A large and apparently growing percentage of us are, according to our own testimony and the standards set by the mainstream healthcare community, overweight. Thus, many of us are compelled to diet and use other strategies to reduce but with apparently only remote chances for long-term weight-loss success. On the other hand, a few of us are not overweight by healthcare standards but are driven to restrict our nutrient intake to an extent that our health becomes jeopardized. Further, Americans are constantly reminded of a connection between eating "healthy foods" and being healthy, slim, and living a long life. Most of us accept the mainstream wisdom, to some degree, that certain foods are "bad," "junk," or "empty calories" (e.g., pie, ice cream, and hamburgers) and are damaging to health and should not be eaten, while other foods are "good, " nutritious, contribute positively to health and longevity, and should be consumed in large amounts (e.g., apples, lettuce, and yogurt). Most people probably assume that our views of "good" and "bad" foods are rooted in sound nutritional science. However, there is strong evidence that the reputation of a specific food can be based to a large extent on that same food's prestige and status before the discovery of vitamins, which occurred in the early twentieth century (this is an issue that will be discussed in the final chapter). Additionally, food reputations have been shaped by many social, historical, and political events of the past 200 years. Thus, the mainstream message that we receive and assimilate about a particular food all too often does not closely correspond with the nutrient content of that same food.[1-5] A potential problem may be that many of us attempt to build our diets with foods that are in good repute but may not be particularly nutritious (e.g., in terms of vitamins and minerals). For instance, it is commonly reported that many of us (and most women) are routinely deficient in certain vitamins and minerals (e.g., iron, calcium, and vitamin C). Further, the perspective that some foods are "good" while others are "bad" for health may make us so extremely anxious about whether to eat and what to eat that the worry itself may cause health problems.

Generally, the intent of this book is not to provide information about the most healthful foods and diets or give advice regarding how people should alter their food consumption. In fact, one could perhaps argue that our bombardment with these sorts of messages, particularly in the past few decades, have contributed to the "good/bad" food viewpoint. Many people are extraordinarily eager to tell others what and how to eat. These messages are often disseminated by legitimate and mainstream sources of nutritional knowledge (government, scientists, nutritionists, dieticians), the food industry, the popular media, as well as many faddish and quackish sources (which may include celebrities). Amazingly, being pretty, slender, and famous can qualify you as a nutrition or exercise expert and gain you an abundance of media attention for stating your opinions on these issues. Although the nutritional messages often vary dramatically, certain portions of the wisdom coming from the mainstream have been fairly consistent for many decades (e.g., apples and other fruits and vegetables are extremely nutritious). So, if the primary goal is not to tell the reader what or how to eat what is the objective? This writing has the following aims. First, to show that foods (e.g., apples) and food nutrients (e.g., dietary fat) have acquired reputations in our culture. These reputations are frequently not well rooted in the best nutritional science and in some cases are legacies from the distant past. The pervasiveness of food reputations, which are too often not in harmony with nutritional facts about foods, suggests widespread confusion about the health value of foods. Further, our reliance on the use of reputations when determining food healthfulness may cause us to make harmful decisions about whether to eat and what to eat and may cause excessive worry and concern about food and eating which may be damaging to health. Second, to provide any information available about the possible origins of food and food-nutrient reputations in

United States history. How did apples become so admired and appreciated in terms of being a healthful food? How did essential nutrients like dietary fat and salt become vilified in our culture and other nutrients like dietary fiber become praised? Third, to indicate (when appropriate) the extreme controversy that exists regarding the healthfulness of our fare. Generally, the goal is to describe food reputations and not contribute to them.

It would be naive to believe that purveyors of nutritional wisdom will reduce or modify the stream of nutritional messages that are called into question in this volume. The best that can be hoped is that this writing will foster a healthy skepticism about the abundance of messages (even those with a mainstream perspective) concerning diet and nutrition that we encounter routinely in our lives and to get more people talking about this issue.

Gender Differences in Views of Food Healthfulness

The notion that people assign status to individual foods has been recognized for well over half a century. Margaret Cussler and Mary de Give writing in early 1950s conveyed the following: people "assign a status to one food, relative to another, much as is done in respect to persons in a society."[6] Anthropologist Carole Counihan concurred and recently asserted that "people endow food with meaning on the basis of its primary qualities." According to Counihan our attitudes concerning a particular food are influenced by many factors including the perceptions of "what it does to the body in terms of weight gain or loss, or feelings of strength or weakness."[7] Counihan, who examined several years' worth of food journals that she had required her college students to keep, conveyed clearly that college students view some foods as "good" and others as "bad" for health. Further, although Counihan did not specifically discuss male and female differences in food journal content, she strongly implied that gender differences concerning attitudes toward foods exist.[8]

Psychologists Mike Oakes and Carole Slotterback have focused more specifically on American's perceptions of healthy and unhealthy foods in both college students and more mature adults. Their approach and goals were different from that of Carole Counihan and others who had examined beliefs about foods. Other investigators had shown previously that women were more concerned about food healthfulness than men and that women eat more "healthy foods"[9, 10] than men. In an attempt to distinguish his research from others, Oakes had this to say: "although other investigators have examined healthy diets and healthy meals and concluded that women (compared to men) and older adults (compared to younger adults) are more knowledgeable and have more healthy eating habits, we are taking a different approach. Our primary goal is to measure and document the confusion regarding what is healthy rather than determine which groups are more knowledgeable or are abiding by the mainstream view of healthy eating."[3] Thus, those who examined attitudes, beliefs, and habits about foods previously, had relied solely on the very same food reputations that are being called into question in this volume. For example, these investigators relied on the mainstream dogma when determining what foods are healthy (i.e., dark breads, rice cakes, apples, grapes, and low-fat milk and cheese). And, if an individual reported knowing that these foods are healthy and eating these sorts of foods mostly, they were judged to be more nutritionally knowledgeable and have healthier eating habits than those who reported eating potatoes and meat. These investigators never really acknowledged any controversy regarding what is healthy and none had considered the notion that men and women may use different information when making decisions concerning what foods are healthy. The research that will be presented below suggests that women (compared to men) view food in a way that agrees with this mainstream perspective. However, it may sometimes be presumptuous and misleading to suggest that one food is healthier than another.

The initial published study that came from this line of inquiry was very simple but unique. College-aged men and women were asked to rate the healthfulness of seventy-two different foods individually on a five-point scale according to how good the food was for them (0 = "very bad" and 4 = "very good"). Previous researchers suggested that women more than men would appreciate both low fat and high vitamin and mineral qualities in foods.[10] Surprisingly, however, in this study foods with high numbers of vitamins and minerals were rated as more healthful by men than by women. Further, women considered low-fat foods with low levels of vitamins and minerals (e.g., Saltine crackers or pretzels) to be equally healthful as low-fat food with high levels of vitamins and minerals (e.g., oatmeal or pasta). Men, on the other hand, generally did not consider low-fat foods with low numbers of vitamins and minerals to be as healthy: they considered low-fat foods more healthful as their vitamin and mineral contents increased. Finally, as expected women (compared to men) considered high-fat foods as less healthy, however, high-fat foods with low numbers of vitamins and minerals (e.g., buttered popcorn or Tostitos) were considered more healthful than high-fat foods with high numbers of vitamins and minerals (e.g., Snickers Bar or hamburgers) and this was observed in both men and women. At first, this seemed very surprising but it probably should not have been given the fact that high-fat foods with lots of vitamins and minerals currently have negative reputations in our society (they are often considered "junk food"). This study was the first to suggest that women consider primarily fat content when determining the healthfulness of foods regardless of the numbers or amounts of other nutrients in the food. Men, on the other hand, considered fat content as well as other nutrients when evaluating food healthfulness.[1] The notion that foods may have reputations concerning healthfulness that do not reflect their nutrient contents was most intriguing. However, for the follow-up study it was necessary to develop an innovative method to examine these food reputations.

Confusion about Food Healthfulness

In this follow-up study college students were once again asked to rate the healthfulness of individual food names (e.g., a potato). Additionally, this time the same students were also asked then to rate the nutrient descriptions of the same foods in terms of healthfulness. The nutrient descriptions contained percentages of the recommended daily value of calories, fat, protein, fiber, cholesterol, and sodium as well as vitamins and minerals in each food. Thus, the students rated the healthfulness of a potato in one part of the survey and the healthfulness of the nutrient description of a potato on another part of the survey. Further, the students had no way of knowing which food description they were rating (i.e., the descriptions were not labeled). The results were amazing, some foods (i.e., their names) clearly had very positive reputations, others had very negative reputations, and very few were considered moderate in terms of healthfulness (see figure 1.1).

Figure 1.1

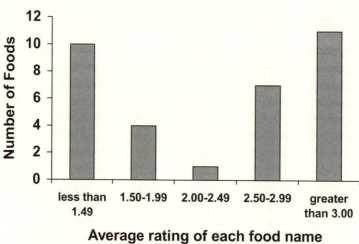

The thirty-three foods names tended to be rated either good for health (i.e., a rating above 2.50) or bad for health (a rating below 1.99) with very few considered moderate for health. Thus, Americans tend to consider foods as either good or bad for health.

Further, the healthfulness rating of a food name (i.e., it's reputation) was frequently very different from the healthfulness rating of the same food's nutrient description (see the table 1.1).[2] A good example of a food with a very positive health reputation (i.e., high name rating) but which had a description health rating that was much lower was the apple. Apples (i.e., the name) were considered very healthful by the students but the nutrient description of apples was not considered particularly healthful. Other foods had more negative reputations (i.e., low name rating) compared to the judgments of their corresponding nutrient descriptions. For example, potatoes were not considered nearly as healthful as their nutrient description. Thus, most foods have reputations and these reputations are often not a clear reflection of the nutrient content of the foods.[2]

Apples were praised by the students in this study because apples get such positive publicity from so many sources. For example, the media generally portrays fruits as being very healthful partially because of their reported high vitamin and mineral content and of

Table 1.1
Mean Ratings of Food Names and Descriptions

	Name Mean (SD)	Descript. Mean (SD)	Paired t- Statistic (E)	Probability less than
No differences between names and descriptions				
1 Egg McMuffin	1.30 (0.88)	1.26 (1.05)	00.43 (.04)	.70
1 hamburger	1.93 (0.77)	2.01 (0.97)	00.73 (.07)	.50
3 oz. tuna in water	3.16 (0.74)	2.97 (0.84)	01.94 (.18)	.06
1 oz. cheese puffs	1.20 (0.65)	1.40 (0.68)	02.59 (.23)	.05
1 raisin bagel	3.03 (0.61)	3.25 (0.68)	02.66 (.24)	.01
1 Big Mac	0.60 (0.68)	0.88 (1.01)	02.54 (.23)	.05
Names rated significantly better than descriptions				
1 cup Cheerios (dry)	3.47 (0.65)	3.18 (0.72)	03.70 (.32)	.001
1 rice cake	2.96 (0.91)	2.13 (0.81)	07.97 (.59)	.001
1 hard boiled egg	2.82 (0.71)	0.57 (0.72)	25.00 (.92)	.001
½ cup Romaine lettuce	3.48 (0.68)	2.56 (0.82)	10.75 (.70)	.001
2 Tbsp. peanut butter	2.11 (0.92)	1.50 (0.82)	05.78 (.47)	.001
1 medium apple	3.56 (0.62)	2.93 (0.76)	06.59 (.52)	.001
1 oz. pretzels	2.76 (0.73)	1.92 (0.77)	08.65 (.62)	.001
8 oz. low-fat Yogurt	3.35 (0.63)	2.95 (0.68)	05.26 (.43)	.001
5 Saltine crackers	2.53 (0.81)	2.01 (0.79)	05.57 (.45)	.001
1 medium carrot	3.65 (0.48)	2.80 (0.82)	10.65 (.70)	.001
1 cup grapes	3.55 (0.55)	2.68 (0.74)	10.98 (.71)	.001
½ cup vanilla ice cream	1.71 (0.72)	1.36 (0.73)	03.78 (.33)	.001
1 beef hotdog	1.29 (0.69)	1.03 (0.65)	03.01 (.27)	.005
1 piece of apple pie	1.61 (0.76)	1.33 (0.71)	02.96 (.26)	.005
1 cup 1 percent fat cot. cheese	2.82 (0.87)	2.41 (1.01)	03.26 (.29)	.005
½ cup applesauce	3.22 (0.71)	2.10 (0.96)	09.55 (.66)	.001
Descriptions rated significantly better than names				
1 glazed donut	0.87 (0.73)	1.63 (0.82)	08.17 (.60)	.001
1 12-oz. beer	1.23 (0.85)	2.26 (0.89)	08.85 (.63)	.001
1 cup pasta	3.16 (0.68)	3.48 (0.63)	04.22 (.36)	.001

	Name Mean (SD)	Descript. Mean (SD)	Paired t- Statistic (E)	Probability less than
Descriptions rated significantly better than names (continued)				
3.5 oz. fried chicken	1.11 (0.84)	1.65 (1.00)	04.73 (.40)	.001
1 oz. potato chips	0.94 (0.64)	2.12 (0.76)	14.43 (.80)	.001
1 Snickers bar	1.03 (0.79)	1.76 (0.80)	07.80 (.58)	.001
1 pkt. apple/cinn oatmeal	3.12 (0.68)	3.35 (0.60)	03.09 (.27)	.005
1 piece beef jerky	1.14 (0.79)	2.08 (0.78)	09.86 (.67)	.001
3.5 cups unbut. popcorn	2.59 (0.79)	3.07 (0.72)	05.31 (.44)	.001
4 gingersnaps	1.83 (0.61)	2.34 (0.64)	06.19 (.49)	.001
1 baked potato w/skin	2.95 (0.82)	3.38 (0.67)	04.60 (.39)	.001

Note. Higher scores indicate greater perceptions of healthiness. (E) indicates effect size, which is expressed as a correlation coefficient.

course "an apple a day keeps the doctor away." However, when the students were confronted with the nutrient description of an apple and the small amounts of vitamins and minerals that apples possess they apparently were not impressed. In this study, it was demonstrated that most fruits and vegetables have a very positive image and that this image is apparently not justified by the food's nutrient contents. Potatoes were an exception, they have a reputation for being fattening, are often considered junk food (e.g., when prepared as French fries), and are not known for their vitamin and mineral contents. In fact, the student respondents generally did not associate the name "potato" with being a vegetable.[2] Possibly even more surprising, articles have been published in reputable journals where the authors did not classify potatoes as vegetables but instead categorized them with red meat. The name "potato" was rated thirteenth (of the thirty-three foods examined in this study) and was considered the least healthful of all the fruits and vegetables on the list. Carrots were rated most healthful of all the food names examined. Yet, the description for a potato reflected high levels of many types of vitamins and minerals as well as respectable amounts of protein and fiber (carrots pale in comparison) and this was reflected in the healthfulness ratings of the potato descriptions. For the food descriptions the potato was considered more healthful than all of the other fruits and vegetables and was rated second overall in terms of healthfulness (just behind pasta). Carrots were rated ninth in the description ratings.[2]

It is noteworthy that according to the primary nutrient table provided by Pennington (1998) a baked potato with skin contains eleven different vitamins and minerals that reach or surpass 10 percent of the daily value for a 2000-calorie diet. An apple, on the other hand, has only one vitamin and no minerals that reach or surpass this standard. And the highly regarded carrot contains only two vitamins and no minerals that reach 10 percent of the daily value. Regarding why Oakes chose 10 percent as a limit rather than 2 percent, which is found on food labels, he had this to say. "The value of 10 percent was chosen as the cut-off to allow for better discrimination among the foods presented. If we had included in our count vitamins and minerals that existed in smaller amounts (i.e., reached or exceeded 2 percent rather than 10 percent) this would have likely hampered our respondents' ability to differentiate foods. For example, according to Pennington (1998), a twelve-ounce beer has at least 2 percent of nine different vitamins and minerals (but none of these reach 10 percent), pasta has at least 2 percent of eleven different vitamins and minerals (and four reach 10 percent or greater). Thus, if 2 percent had been used food items with very small amounts of many vitamins and minerals (e.g., "beer") would appear to be similar, in vitamin and mineral content, to foods with large amounts of many vitamins and minerals (e.g., "pasta")."[2]

Although the reputations of individual foods like apples and potatoes will be discussed in a more historical context in the final chapter, for now hopefully it will suffice to convey that the students' ratings of potatoes (i.e., the name) reflect a negative historical legacy as well as more recent bad press directed at the unpretentious spud. For example, nutritional researchers from prestigious Harvard University recently related, "You want to eat minimal amounts of pasta, for example, or potatoes, things that are just starches and don't have much else going for them."[11] Even the1972 *World Book Encyclopedia* indicated that potatoes had a reputation for being fattening.[12] Further, the popularity of the term "couch potato" probably contributes to the unwholesome reputation of potatoes as being nutritionally insignificant and promoters of obesity. Potatoes are composed primarily of complex carbohydrates and are now getting battered by both the mainstream low-fat enthusiasts (who generally praise complex carbohydrates) and the upstart low-carbohydrate advocates. Both groups seem to see potatoes as fattening and with little nutritional value. Potatoes apparently have more essential nutrients than most people (including most authorities) think; they are clearly one of the most nutritious vegetables in terms of vitamin and mineral content. However, different from most other vegetables and according to the United States Department of Agriculture, fresh potato consumption has declined in the United States over the past thirty years or so.[13] Those in the low-carbohydrate camp clearly see potatoes as contributing to obesity and disease (e.g., diabetes and heart disease). Surprisingly, pasta, which has received extreme praise by mainstream health reporters over the years and is in the ground floor of the government's food pyramid, is now being criticized by many for the same reasons. Foods like potatoes and pasta are thought to be too easily digested and thus, cause extreme spikes in blood sugar levels, which according to one hypothesis is conducive to overeating, obesity, and disease.

Finally, the students (especially the women) assessed the food names using a mainstream approach to food healthfulness (e.g., fruits and vegetables are good and meat is bad) but the mainstream theme regarding food healthfulness was much less evident in the assessments of food descriptions (compare figures 1.1 and 1.2). Also one thing that was abundantly clear from this study was that the primary predictor (and the only predictor for women) concerning whether a food (i.e., it's name) would be rated as healthful or unhealthful was the food's fat content. Thus, fat content was considered the most important characteristic when evaluating the healthfulness of foods by both men and women.[2] It should be no surprise to any of us that television, newspaper, and magazine coverage of nutritional issues has been shown to be dominated by information about dietary fat at the expense of other nutrients. The terms low-fat, reduced fat, non-fat, and of course fat-free have become synonymous for good for you, nutritious, and healthy and this research suggests that this is especially true for young women.

There were also interesting differences evident between men and women in this study. The discrepancy between the health ratings of a particular food (i.e., the food's name) and that same food's nutrient description was generally greater for women than men. These gender differences were due to the fact that women rated the

Figure 1.2

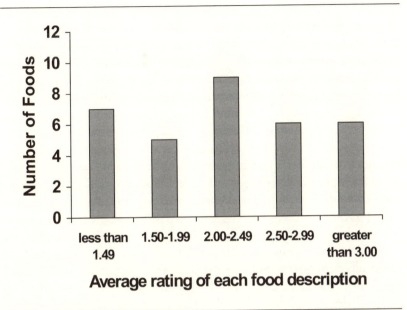

The average ratings for the thirty-three food descriptions were scattered much more evenly than for the food name ratings. Thus, the food descriptions were not considered as good or bad for health, in fact, many were viewed as moderate for health.

food names differently than men (description ratings were always similar for men and women). The most probable explanation for this is that women are more often than men the target of health and nutrition information (in, for example, magazines) and thus are more routinely bombarded and overloaded with such information.[1] Thus, food reputations have become somewhat more important and influential to women than men. For example, women (compared to men) considered carrots very healthful but the healthfulness ratings of men and women for the nutrient descriptions of carrots were much lower and did not vary.[2] Thus, carrots have a very positive reputation (especially for women) but this reputation is apparently not justified by the nutrient content of carrots. Further, women considered only the fat contents of foods (i.e., food names) when evaluating the food's healthfulness; men, on other hand, considered both fat content and amounts of vitamins and minerals. These results strongly suggest that women have assimilated stronger biases about foods than have men and these biases primarily involve the mainstream media's vilification of dietary fat. These biases about foods, which are often not based on the food's nutrient content (other than levels of fat), likely cause us to make poor decisions regarding what to purchase and eat.[2] For example, it may be harmful if we are eating large quantities of apples and lettuce instead of more nutrient-dense foods because we believe these products to be loaded with vitamins and minerals. Foods with good reputations are sometimes not as nutritionally sound as those with poorer reputations. Certainly, it has been reported that some Americans (particularly women) consume lower than recommended amounts of calories, which places them at risk for nutritional deficiencies[14] and other dangers. Further, most women in the United States do not get the recommended levels of minerals such as iron and calcium.[15]

One other point should be made regarding these two studies, college women tended to convey that foods such as rice cakes and unbuttered popcorn were healthy foods. When asked why they rated these foods as they did the women often related because they "fill up the stomach, " are "filling, " or some similar comment. Thus, foods with low levels of vitamins and minerals are often praised as being healthful by women because it is assumed that they satisfy the appetite.[2] However, the extent to which low nutrient foods like rice cakes and unbuttered popcorn quell hunger is debatable.

Several replications of this name/description study using more mature adults (e.g., people above age twenty-five) as participants have since been published and very similar results were found. Thus, the use of food reputations when assessing the healthfulness of foods is pervasive in our society among adults of all ages.[3-5] Americans seem to be somewhat confused about the nutritional aspects of our foods.

One other illustration addressing the issue of gender differences in perception of foods involved asking college students a simple question. Which has a greater number of vitamins and minerals an apple (which has a very positive reputation) or a Big Mac (which has a very negative reputation)? In truth these two are not even close in terms of levels of vitamins and minerals, a Big Mac has significant amounts of many vitamins and minerals (thirteen) and apples have one (vitamin C). However, more than 80 percent of the students indicated that an apple has more vitamins and minerals than a Big Mac. Further, college women were significantly more likely than men to relate that an apple had more vitamins and minerals than the Big Mac.[16] This should not be surprising: we have assimilated the view that fast food is unhealthful and that Big Macs are "junk food, " a term typically reserved for foods perceived to be low in nutrients (not including fat and calories). Some reform-minded citizens are now advocating government taxation of this perceived "junk food" as a way to keep Americans from eating it. Interestingly, it may be a sign of the times that one gentleman recently filed a law suit in the city of New York against four fast-food chains because he claims that they made him unhealthy and fat. The lawyer for the complainant has indicated that his goal is social reform concerning fast food consumption.

Paul Rozin from the University of Pennsylvania has also explored American beliefs about foods. Rozin and his colleagues have shown that many Americans tend to view certain foods or food nutrients as poisons and that even trace levels of fat, salt, beef, sugar, or chocolate are viewed by many as being harmful to health. Rozin also found that only one half of his respondents indicated that a diet free of mercury is healthier than the same diet with a pinch of mercury. Similarly, about one half of his respondents related that a diet free of salt or fat is healthier than the same calorie diet with a teaspoon of salt or fat per day. However, it is important to understand that mercury exposure is extremely toxic (in fact deadly) and any mercury exposure should be avoided: on the other hand, salt and fat are essential for life and a teaspoon per day of either salt or fat is well within our basic nutritional requirements. Further, when Rozin and colleagues asked people which food from a list including corn, alfalfa sprouts, hot dogs, spinach, peaches, bananas, or milk chocolate could support life for a single year most of the respondents indicated bananas (42 percent of the respondents) followed by spinach (27 percent of the respondents). These are both foods that currently have very good reputations in our society but are actually low in nutrients necessary for survival. According to Rozin and coworkers, animal products are generally more nutritious and would be most likely to contain the necessary nutrients for survival. Thus, the foods most likely to support life for a year would be (believe or not) hot dogs (only 4 percent of the respondents said this) or possibly milk chocolate (only 3 percent of the respondents conveyed this).[17] Of course, hot dogs and milk chocolate are viewed negatively in terms of healthfulness, thus, most of the respondents did not consider them appropriate answers.

A Generous Helping of Exaggeration and Contradiction

It has been argued that the healthfulness (or lack of healthfulness) of some food nutrients get exaggerated at the expense of other nutrients.[18] Similarly, much of the information we get regarding food nutrition is incomplete because those who disseminate nutritional messages too often emphasize just certain nutrient characteristics of foods (e.g., the levels of fat and cholesterol) and ignore others. Further, many consumers perceive extreme contradictions in the advice we get about food. Most foods get predominantly good press or mostly bad press (which may in part explain figure 1.1). However, a few foods seem to flop around on the good/bad continuum or their qualities are debated by the purveyors of nutritional wisdom. Dairy products are a good example, they have a wholesome reputation to some extent. However, dairy products have received some bad press over the years. One milk maligning book from a few years back mocked the wisdom of Dear Old Mom by warning us in its title, *"Don't Drink Your Milk: New Frightening Medical Facts About the World's Most Overrated Nutrient."* In this volume it was stated unequivocally that milk should be consumed only by cows and numerous potential health problems with humans consuming cow's milk were cited (e.g., allergies and digestive problems).[19] Eggs also have a wholesome reputation. The popular media has praised eggs repeatedly over the past several decades because they are often perceived to have an abundance of nutrients. However, at the same time eggs have been receiving negative press for the past fifty years primarily due to their cholesterol content.[20] It seems that eggs have made somewhat of a comeback in recent years primarily because it has been reported that dietary cholesterol probably has very little impact on blood cholesterol for most people. Apparently the bad press about eggs has captured the public's attention most because egg consumption among Americans dropped drastically throughout most of the last half of the twentieth century but rose slightly in 1998 and 1999.[13] The manufacturers of butter and margarine have been feuding ever since margarine was patented in 1873 and first produced three years later in the United States.[21] For many years experts touted the health advantages of margarine over butter, however, butter has gotten the upper hand lately due to the fact that certain components in margarine (i.e., trans-fatty acids) have been reported by some to have particularly negative effects on blood cholesterol.[22] This negative press concerning the dangers of margarine apparently is beginning to be assimilated by the American public. Margarine use has declined recently among Americans but butter consumption continues to show a consistent decline and is less than half what it was in the 1950s.[13]

Food Stereotypes

When we hear a few negative comments about a food we tend to get an overall negative attitude about the food in a way that goes well beyond the original negative messages. One good example is the Big Mac, no one knowledgeable about nutrition has commented that Big Macs are low in vitamins and minerals. However, since we often hear negative commentary about the fat content of the Big Mac and due to the poor reputation of fast food in general we may actually remember information about Big Macs that no knowledgeable person ever actually said, that being that they have low levels of vitamins and minerals (we have a stereotype about Big Macs). Drugs also have reputations. After hearing the abundant negative press about the drug heroin throughout their lives, college students assimilate the notion that heroin is the worst on every measure of drug harmfulness. Thus, when asked about which drug has the most deadly withdrawal symptoms the answer usually is "heroin." However, all of the textbooks for the course convey that nobody ever dies of heroin withdrawal and that alcohol has much more life threatening withdrawal symptoms. Thus, we have stereotypes about drugs that do not entirely agree with medical facts.[23]

Further, as alluded to previously, it is not uncommon for media sources to exaggerate the risk of eating certain foods. For example, it is generally accepted now that the Alar/apple threat of ten-fifteen years ago was generally overstated[24] and may have done more harm than good. Also, the overall vilification of dietary fat may well be inappropriate given the scientific controversy concerning its danger and what appears to be (at most) a minute risk to the individual. For example, many scientists as well as those from the food industry are now advising Americans to eat some types of fat to benefit our health (e.g., Omega-3 fatty acids). Additionally, Paul Rozin has suggested that people are generally poorly equipped to handle information about very low risk activities.[25] As a consequence, many of us may overemphasize the dangers that we hear about foods and overreact by restricting the variety of foods that we eat, a tendency which may be unhealthy. Thus, as it concerns food, low-risk activities often get exaggerated by those giving information and those receiving information. The notion that exaggeration of risk may impact food reputations does not in any way imply that legitimate concerns about our food supply do not exist.

Are Americans Overly Concerned about Food?

There is also speculation that the stress and worry regarding consumption of essential dietary nutrients that have gained negative reputations may have deleterious effects to our health. Paul Rozin organized a cross-cultural study and showed that Americans worry about their diet more than the other cultures that were examined (i.e., Belgium, France, and Japan) and get less pleasure from their food. Further, people from the United States tend to select more modified foods for consumption (e.g., more low-fat foods). However, Americans perceive themselves to be unhealthy eaters compared to those from the other countries. People from France were typically on the other extreme compared to the Americans, that is, they were less worried, received more pleasure from food, and used fewer modified products. Generally, across all cultures, women tended to report being more worried and concerned about food and to modify their diets more than did men. In fact, men were described as being more like the French (pleasure oriented) and women more like Americans (negative/health oriented). It is also important to mention that it has been frequently reported that the French consume more dietary fat (including saturated fat) and smoke more than Americans, yet, heart disease is much less prevalent in France compared to the United States (often referred to as "the French paradox"). The implication provided by Rozin and his colleagues is that extreme worry about food may have negative effects on our health and our length of life. Further, the government and nutrition experts should consider the possible hazards to promoting dietary changes, how difficult long-term dietary changes tend to be, the cost of failure, and the proposed benefits.[26] The controversy surrounding the health benefits of reducing levels of fat, cholesterol, and sodium in our diets will be discussed in later chapters.

From Fat to Fresh?

Surveys of nutritional habits and concerns have typically revealed that dietary fat was the number one nutrition concern of Americans in the 1990s. Throughout the 1990s it was not uncommon for surveys to indicate that the majority of shoppers were checking nutritional labels for fat content and trying to reduce their fat consumption.[18] Further, many shoppers reported that the fat content on nutritional labels influenced their purchasing decisions.[27] However, this may be changing slightly, at least for more mature adults. For better or worse, a recent survey found that "freshness" was as important as the "fat content" of food when determining food healthfulness, at least among Northeastern Pennsylvania grocery shoppers. Shoppers were asked at local grocery stores to select the food characteristic most important for healthfulness from a list that was provided. The options were "calorie content, " "natural/unprocessed, " "vitamin/mineral content, " "freshness, " "sodium content, " "fat content, " and "protein content." Shoppers who reported dieting, regardless of whether they were men or women, generally indicated that "fat content" was the most important characteristic of food healthfulness. Non-dieting shoppers (of both sexes) typically related that "freshness" was the most important health characteristic to them. However, it appears that the majority of college-aged women, regardless of dieting status, are still extremely preoccupied with the fat content of food more than any other food characteristic.[28]

It recently has been reported that some people are weary of hearing what foods they should eat and are becoming somewhat more cautious and skeptical about dietary recommendations, particularly as they involve dietary fat. Yet, this viewpoint is apparently not widespread. Those of us who are skeptical about nutritional advice tend to be younger (ages eighteen to thirty-five) and older (ages sixty-plus) adults, but less so for middle-aged people who apparently are more comfortable with dietary recommendations. Men and those of lower socioeconomic status are also somewhat more likely to view current nutritional wisdom with some skepticism.[29]

Men, low socioeconomic status individuals, and perhaps even the elderly were probably more resistant to this mainstream message to begin with.

Names in Food Advertising

Marion Nestle[30] recently wrote a very thorough description of the extreme influence of the food industry on dietary advice coming from our federal government. However, for this discussion the manipulation of names and enticing words by advertisers, who are intent on convincing us that their products are healthy, will be emphasized.

If a particular food has a negative reputation and if this reputation is potentially reducing sales the producers or manufacturers may change the name of the food. For example, what used to be known as Super Sugar Crisp now sounds a bit more healthful with the moniker Golden Crisp, Sugar Smacks are now just Smacks, Corn Pops were once Sugar Corn Pops, prunes are now dried plums, and Salted Nut Roll was changed to Nut Roll. Also, Frosted Flakes were once advertised as Sugar Frosted Flakes. Additionally, the not so wholesome sounding cereal names Sugar Jets and Twinkies, (both were General Mills products) and Sugar Frosted Chex (from Ralston Purina) also have undergone name changes or are no longer available.[31] Finally, the initials KFC seem to be preferred now by advertisers over the name Kentucky Fried Chicken.

The terms organic, natural, and fresh are common on food labels nowadays: these terms give the consumer an impression that these foods are healthful alternatives. However, according to the Food and Drug Administration (FDA) and the United States Department of Agriculture (USDA) there are no regulations or standards that limit the use of the terms natural or fresh on food labels. The term natural on a food label does not mean that the food has no additives, preservatives, or artificial substances. Even if "natural" did mean that there was nothing artificial in the product it still would not be synonymous with healthful or safe. As mentioned before the concept of freshness is considered to be a very positive characteristic of food these days, however, it certainly does not mean that the product was recently packaged, prepared, or harvested. There is apparently one exception at least for poultry: the term "fresh" on the label of a poultry product means that the product has never been frozen solid[32] (ironically, a chicken could be spoiled and yet be fresh). This idea, i.e., that fresh is more healthful than frozen, dates back to the early twentieth century when freezing was done primarily to preserve foods that were already beginning to spoil.[33] Perhaps the reputation of frozen food has improved, today frozen foods are not considered to be unsafe or nutritionally unsound. For example Ruth Yaron who wrote *Super Baby Food* did not distinguish between fresh and frozen foods regarding nutritional contents but indicated that nutritionally speaking both are preferred over canned products when making baby food.[34] Thus, the terms "natural" and "fresh" on food labels often do not translate into healthy, safe, and nutritious.

Starting back in October of 1993 the term "organic" on a food label became more meaningful. For a food to be labeled as organic it must now meet certain food production and handling standards set by the United States Department of Agriculture (USDA). For example, products produced on organic farms are inspected periodically for pesticides, non-organic residue, and toxins (e.g., arsenic and lead). Further, there are limitations on the types of fertilizers that can be used on organically labeled foods. Dairy herds and other livestock must be provided organically produced feed (at least primarily). The use of "plastic pellets" for roughage in livestock feed is not allowed as well as "manure refeeding." Livestock cannot be given growth promoters, hormones, or antibiotics for any reason; however, vaccines are allowed to keep animals healthy. Sick or injured animals must be treated but if treated with prohibited medication they cannot be sold as organic. Organically raised livestock must be given access to the outdoors, this includes pasture time so that the animals can graze. A grocery store product can be labeled as "100 percent organic" if it contains only organically produced ingredients. Foods that are mostly organic (i.e., at least 95 percent organic ingredients) can be labeled "organic." If a food has 70 percent organic ingredients the label can indicate "made with organic ingredients, " however, foods with less than 70 percent organic ingredients cannot use the terms organic on the primary display panel but can indicate the specific ingredients that are organically produced in the ingredients statement.[35] Is a "100 percent organic" product more nutritious than non-organic alternatives? Most authorities would say no, fertilizer increases yield but does not influence the nutritional content of the foods produced. Nutrition content depends more on the genetics of the plant, climate, maturity when harvested, and "freshness" when consumed.[36-40] However, it is likely that organic farming methods do promote and preserve the fertility of the soil and may foster more humane treatment of livestock. There may also be a smaller likelihood of potentially dangerous chemicals in these products.

Food manufacturers often change the ingredients in their products in order for the products to sound more healthful or at least emphasize (on the label) the characteristics of their products that have positive reputations (e.g., when licorice packages indicate that the product is fat free). Before the Nutrition Labeling and Education Act (NLEA) of 1990, food manufacturers were sometimes deceptive about manipulating the public's view of their products. The NLEA provided many important reforms in food labeling, for example, the act required that serving sizes be standardized so that a particular food manufacturer could not decide on their own what the serving size would be for their products. Before the NLEA, if a product had high amounts of a nutrient with a negative reputation (e.g., fat) the manufacturer would manipulate the serving size (i.e., make it smaller) so that the product appeared to have less fat per serving.[27]

What is labeled and advertised as "wheat bread" is made primarily with ordinary enriched white flour (which of course comes from wheat). Brown breads at the grocery store with the term "wheat" on the label have enriched white flour as their primary ingredient. The brown color (which is created with caramel coloring used to make it look brown and nutritious) and the term "wheat" on the label convey healthfulness to most of us but these are not made from whole grain flour (at least not primarily). Further, products advertised as consisting of many grains (e.g., "nine grain bread") are also made primarily from enriched white flour. If you want whole wheat or whole grain bread it should have the term "whole" on the label. Whether whole-wheat flour is more healthful than enriched white flour can be debated, however, 100 percent whole-wheat flour has more protein, fat, fiber, and vitamins and minerals than enriched white flour.

Primitive versions of white flour have been available for hundreds of years, however, about 150 years ago steel rollers were developed in Europe and adopted in the United States that would not only grind the grain but also separate the components (e.g., the bran and endosperm). This made white flour more abundant and less expensive.[41] Before the twentieth century, white flour was associated with social status and was consumed primarily by the wealthy: it would have been considered a rare treat for a farm family. Most people considered white flour superior to the more primitive and ordinary dark flour.[42] White flour was considered superior for several reasons: (1) its whiteness was symbolic of purity and wholesomeness; (2) the texture of white bread is lighter and makes crisper toast; (3) many sources say that white flour keeps longer; and (4) wholegrain bread requires more skill and time to make.[43] Some people still object to the use of steel rollers when making flour (even wholegrain flour) on the basis that the metal itself or the extreme heat generated by the steel rollers damages the flour. Stone ground, wholegrain flour is preferred by those who take their baked goods very seriously.[41]

Although there are many types of sugars, as alluded to earlier when describing the removal of the word "sugar" in breakfast cereal names, the term "sugar" generally has a negative image as it pertains to food ingredients. White sugar has been rumored to cause a variety of afflictions such as arthritis, cancer, mental illness, hemorrhoids, varicose veins, hair loss, impotence, scurvy as well as vitamin and mineral deficiencies, obesity, crime, drug addiction, and suicide.[44, 45] These rumors ultimately contributed to the use of highly revered terms like "sugar free, " "less, " and "light" on food labels. Honey, on the other hand, has a more positive image and the presence of honey in a product is frequently billed as a positive characteristic on food labels. Interestingly, however, any differences in vitamin and mineral levels in these two sweeteners is miniscule and not worth mentioning (they both have virtually none).[46] If you're interested in obtaining vitamins and minerals from sweeteners maple sugar (although expensive) is slightly better than honey, and brown sugar (which is a mixture of white sugar and molasses) is better yet. Probably, the biggest difference in nutrient amounts between honey and white sugar concerns their calorie contents. A tablespoon of honey has about 30 percent more calories than a tablespoon of white sugar.[47] However, honey is more sweet than sugar and less honey may be needed. Finally, much of what has been rumored about white sugar apparently is not true. For example honey (which is mostly sugar itself) may promote tooth decay more than does white sugar[47] and the best evidence indicates that sugar does not make kids hyperactive.[48]

Summary and Concluding Remarks

Thus, common foods have acquired reputations or stereotypes in terms of healthfulness that are often not congruent with their nutrient contents. The main food component (and probably the only component for most women) on which a food's health reputation is based is the food's fat content at the expense of other essential nutrients. Women, who likely are more bombarded with nutritional messages than men, are influenced and guided more by food reputations than are men. Further, Paul Rozin has indicated that trace amounts of some foods (e.g., beef) are considered unhealthful by many people and even small amounts of essential food nutrients (i.e., salt and fat) are often considered toxic components of foods. Some of our beliefs concerning the healthfulness of our fare appear to be food status legacies from the nineteenth and early twentieth centuries (a topic that will be discussed more in the final chapter). Other beliefs about our sustenance have been acquired more recently from those in the food industry, recognized nutritional authorities, the government, celebrities, and the popular press. A food's reputation is shaped not only by its nutritional characteristic but also by an array of social, historical, cultural, and political factors. Our current views of foods and food nutrients may take much of the pleasure from eating and contribute to unnecessary worry and concern, malnutrition, and poor dietary habits that may be conducive to eating disorders and possibly obesity. In the next chapter, attempts will be made to show how historical events and personalities of the distant and recent past have for better or worse impacted our beliefs about foods.

Notes

1. M. E. Oakes and C. S. Slotterback, Gender differences in perceptions of the healthiness of foods, *Psychology and Health* 16 (2001[a]), 57-65.
2. M. E. Oakes and C. S. Slotterback, What's in a name? A comparison of men's and women's judgements about food names and their nutrient contents, *Appetite* 36 (2001[b]), 29-40.
3. M. E. Oakes and C. S. Slotterback, Judgements of food healthfulness: food name stereotypes in adults over age 25, *Appetite* 37 (2001[c]), 1-8.
4. M. E. Oakes, Differences in Judgments of Food Healthfulness by Young and Elderly Women, *Food Quality and Preference* 14 (2003), 227-236.
5. M. E. Oakes, An examination of the influence of gender and dieting status on ratings of food healthfulness. In S. P. Anderson, ed.: *Advances in psychology research 16* (New York: Nova Science Publishers 2002).

6. M. Cusslerand M. L. de Give, Twixt the cup and the lip (New York: Twayne Publishers 1952). p. 152
7. C. M. Counihan, *The anthropology of food and body: Gender, meaning, and power* (New York: Routledge 1999). p. 114
8. Counihan, *The anthropology of food and body*: p. 115
9. L. Rappoport, G. R. Peters, R. Downey, T. McCann, and L. Huff-Corzine, Gender and age differences in food cognition, *Appetite* 20 (1993), 33-52.
10. M. K. Hunt, D. J. McNamara, K. Glanz, J. R. Herbert, C. Probart, G. Sorensen, S. Thomas, M. L. Hixson, L. Linnan, and R. Palombo, Measures of food choice behavior related to intervention messages in worksite health promotion, *Journal of Nutritional Education* 29 (1997), 3-11.
11. CNN.com—Elizabeth Cohen: The Skinny on 'good fats'—July 8, 2002: Http// www.cnn.com/2002/HE...fitness/07/08/cohen.fat.otsc/index.ht
12. Field Enterprises Educational Corporation. (1973) *World Book Encyclopedia*. (Chicago, IL: Author).
13. USDA, Agriculture Fact Book 2000.
14. B. J. Rolls, I. C. Fedoroff, and J. F. Guthrie, Gender differences in eating behavior and body weight regulation, *Health Psychology* 10 (1991), 133-142.
15. S. A. French and R. W. Jeffery, Consequences of dieting to lose weight effects on physical and mental health, *Health Psychology* 13 (1994), 195-212.
16. M. E. Oakes, unpublished data
17. P. Rozin, M. Ashmore, and M. Markwith, Lay American conceptions of nutrition: Dose insensitivity, categorical thinking, contagion, and the monotonic mind, *Health Psychology* 15 (1996), 438-447.
18. N. E. Schwartz and S. T. Borra, What do consumers really think about dietary fat? *Journal of the American Dietetic Association* 97 (1997), S73-S75.
19. F. A. Oski, *Don't drink your milk! New frightening medical facts about the world's most overrated nutrient* (Syracuse, NY: Mollica 1983).
20. W. A. McIntosh, The symbolism of eggs in American culture: A sociological analysis, *Journal of the American College of Nutrition* 19 (2000), 532S-539S.
21. I. D. Garard, *The story of food* (Westport, CT: The AVI Publishing Company, Inc. 1974)
22. G. J. Nelson, Dietary fat, trans-fatty acids, and risk of coronary heart disease, *Nutritional Reviews* 56 (1998), 250-252.
23. M. E. Oakes, *Changing drug stereotypes*. Poster presented at the ninth annual APS institute on the teaching of psychology, American Psychological Society meeting , New Orleans, LA.
24. S. Gebo, *What's left to eat?* (New York: McGraw Hill, Inc. 1992).
25. P. Rozin, Disorders of food selection: The compromise of pleasure, *Annals of the New York Academy of Sciences* 575 (1989), 376-385.
26. P. Rozin, C. Fischler, S. Imada, A. Sarubin, and A. Wrzesniewski, Attitudes to food and the role of food in life in the U.S.A., Japan, Flemish Belgium and France: Possible implications for the diet-health debate, *Appetite,* 33 (1999), 163-180.
27. L. S. Sims, *The politics of fat* (Armonk, NY: M. E. Sharpe 1998).
28. M. E. Oakes and C. S. Slotterback, The good, the bad, and the ugly: Characteristics used by young, middle-aged, and older men and women, dieters and non-dieters to judge the healthfulness of foods, *Appetite* 38 (2002), 91-97.
29. R. E. Patterson, J. A. Satia, A. R. Kristal, M. L. Neuhouser, and A. Drewnowski, Is there a consumer backlash against the diet and health message, *Journal of the American Dietetic Association* 101 (2001), 37-41.
30. M. Nestle, *Food politics: How the food industry influences nutrition and health* (Berkeley: University of California Press 2002).

31. J. Rosenthal, Hunger expert says many dry cereals are not nutritious, *New York Times* (Friday, July 24, 1970).
32. http://www.fsis.usda.gov
33. H. Levenstein, *Paradox of plenty: A social history of eating in modern America* (New York: Oxford University Press 1993), 106.
34. R. Yaron, *Super baby food* (Archibald, PA: F. J. Roberts Publishing Company 2000).
35. *http://www.ams.usda.gov*
36. E.M. Whelan, and F. J. Stare, *The one-hundred-percent natural, purely organic, cholesterol free, megavitamin, low carbohydrate nutrition hoax* (New York: Atheneum 1983), 138-139.
37. V. Herbert, and S. Barrett, *Vitamins and "health" foods: The great American hustle* (Philadelphia, PA: George F. Stickley Company 1981), 112.
38. J. V. Young, *The medical messiahs: A social history of health quackery in twentieth-century America* (Princeton, New Jersey: Princeton University Press 1967), 351.
39. M. Castleman, The myth and promise of organic produce. *Medical Self-Care,* fall (1981).
40. Levenstein, *Paradox of plenty:* 163.
41. A. Davidson, *The Oxford companion to food* (New York: Oxford University Press 1999).
42. E. N. McIntosh, *American food habits in historical perspective* (Westport, CT: Praeger 1995).
43. R. W. Lacy, *Hard to swallow: A brief history of food* (New York: Cambridge University Press 1994).
44. W. Dufty, *Sugar Blues* (New York: Warner Book 1975) p. 183.
45. J. Yudkin, *Sweet and dangerous* (New York: Peter H. Wyden, Inc. 1972).
46. J. A. T. Pennington, *Bowes and Church's Food values of portions commonly used* (Philadelphia, PA: Lippincott 1998).
47. R. Rosauer, Sweet and good, good and sweet, *Total Fitness* March (1983).
48. W. Bennett, The taste that failed, *American Health* July/August (1983).

2

We Are What We Eat

Early Health Gurus

Although dietary fat and cholesterol from animal flesh was likely no more a concern for them than any other ingredient found in meat, the first persons to publicly eschew consumption of dietary animal lipids in the United States were a small group of immigrants who came from England to the United States in the early nineteenth century and who espoused vegetarianism. Their reasons for emphasizing the importance of vegetarianism came primarily from the Bible. Several Bible passages suggest that killing animals might be inappropriate but most interesting (for the current purpose) was the fact that consumption of animal flesh (according to the Bible) may cause us to "stumble or offend" and become "riotous."[1] The notion that meat had stimulant properties and could cause us to make bad decisions concerning sexual behavior and aggression was alive and well throughout the nineteenth and twentieth centuries. Thus, although moral convictions and sympathy for animals was very influential to these early American vegetarians, health issues were also important. Digestive problems, or as it was called then, "dyspepsia" (or even "Americanitis")[2] became more common in the nineteenth century and meat was thought to be major contributor to this discomfort. In addition to what we ate, how we ate also likely had an impact on our digestive woes. It's often assumed that the pace of American eating has increased and that American table manners have deteriorated over the past few decades, and perhaps they have. However, Carson described accounts of nineteenth-century American table manners in the following way. Americans tend to eat all they want and the mode of eating was "not delicate."[3] Our ancestors apparently tended to "gobble, gulp, and go."[4] Further, Carson indicated that no ceremony was observed; "every man for himself, and none for his neighbor; hurrying, snatching, gulping like famished wildcats; victuals disappearing as if by magic."[5]

Probably the most notable of these early advocates of dietary change was the man from which the Graham cracker received its name. William Sylvester Graham (1794-1851) was a Presbyterian minister and self-styled physician who advocated a diet of fresh vegetables, fruits, and whole-grain bread. He denounced the consumption of meat, salt, and spices, as well as the white bread of his day (although it was not nearly as processed as today's white bread) and favored the consumption of fresh fruits and vegetables in their raw form. Additionally, as you might expect he also came down hard against tobacco, alcohol, and sex. Graham was ardent and verbose about his dietary reform as well as his religion and he was apparently uninhibited in his preaching about these convictions. In short, although he had some followers many of which came after his death, many people of his day considered him arrogant, fanatical, irrational, and a bit of a nuisance.[1] Interestingly, although Graham did not receive overwhelming support with the general public in his lifetime his influence is very evident today: first, he was probably the first advocate of bran consumption; second, he stressed the benefits of exercise as a means to maintain health and as an antidote to disease; third, he, in part, inspired the breakfast cereal movement; fourth, he was the first person to publicly accuse food manufacturers of adulterating their products for profit (e.g., Graham criticized the fact that bakers were adding substances like chalk and clay to their flour); fifth, he was really the first person to publicly praise the importance of natural and fresh foods; and sixth, he clearly felt that red meat contained harmful ingredients and that salt was detrimental to health and aroused sexual desires. According to Graham, meat aroused more basic and primitive drives and caused a desire to drink liquor (meat was usually salted in those days). Thus, meat should be avoided. Graham felt that meat consumption enhanced sexual desire, and sexual activity of any kind (but particularly masturbation) was unhealthful. Masturbation was thought to cause many health problems ranging from nervousness to blindness, stupidity, and insanity.[6] A strict adherence to Graham's dietary regimen would quell tendencies toward masturbation and if that didn't quiet the libido Graham recommended trying handcuffs. Interestingly, he also frowned on extensive schooling: too much book learning was thought to cripple the nervous system.[7]

Graham would likely be squirming in his grave if he knew the primary ingredients in today's Graham crackers. Today's Graham crackers have white enriched flour as their primary ingredient with sugar as the second most abundant ingredient. Graham flour, which is another name for whole-wheat flour, is often the third most common ingredient and would have met with William Sylvester's approval.

Graham had a direct influence on John Harvey Kellogg. Kellogg was a physician and Seventh Day Adventist who is most noted for his contribution to ready-to-eat breakfast cereal, however, he was not the first to develop a type of cold breakfast cereal. The first cold cereal breakfast was developed by James A. Jackson several years earlier (in 1863) and was called Granula (it was an ancestor of Grape Nuts). Similar to Grape Nuts, Jackson's product was extremely hard and dry and the preferred method of preparation involved soaking Granula overnight in water and milk. Thus, it was not an instant breakfast. Shredded wheat was the next installment in breakfast cereal evolution (invented in the early 1890s) but was not a Kellogg product. Rather, it was created by a man named Henry Perky who was working out of Denver. Corn flakes were first manufactured by Kellogg in 1898 and improved in the early 1900s.

Breakfast for most Americans in 1876 (the year that Kellogg was hired as chief physician at Battle Creek, Michigan) was built around fried potatoes and salted meat. Breakfast cereal was first marketed as a more healthful and bowel-friendly (i.e., easily digestible) alternative to the fatty and salty fare of the late nineteenth century. In his day Kellogg was known for much more than just his influence on breakfast food, he was probably the major health guru of his day[1]. In addition to advocating much of the dietary reform first proposed by Graham, he also endorsed hydrotherapy which involved baths of all sorts (i.e., hot, cold, steam, or even salt baths), showers, douches, fomentations, and devices called the wet girdle and cold mitten. The inward areas also benefited from water, he advocated the consumption of vegetable teas and herbs but considered cola drinks (which were advertised as being healthful in those days) a form of "insidious poison." And if those teas weren't stimulating enough Kellogg could pump fifteen gallons of water through your bowels in a matter of minutes with his high-powered enema machine. Electricity, massage (often using gizmos that would pummel, shake, pound, and vibrate you), medical gymnastics, laughing exercises, dancing, and frequent changes of underwear were other therapeutic techniques used by Dr. Kellogg and his colleagues at Battle Creek, Michigan in the late nineteenth and early twentieth century.[7] Kellogg also emphasized the immoral, indecent, and aggressive behavior brought on by consuming meat as well as its tendencies to elicit dyspepsia and contribute to aging and degenerative disease.

Parenthetically, it is noteworthy that Doctor Kellogg frowned on sugar consumption and would likely be appalled by the use of this ingredient in the manufacture of many of today's breakfast cereals. Also, Kellogg considered easily digestible foods to be beneficial to health: dyspepsia is often mentioned as a major health problem during this time period. However, these sorts of complaints were probably somewhat trendy in those days among the middle and upper classes.[8] Ironically, although foods that could be digested easily were praised for their healthfulness in those days, as mentioned previously the idea in favor these days is that easily digestible foods cause health problems. Finally, before fortification boosted their nutrient levels, cereals like Corn Flakes were quite low in vitamins and minerals and probably were not a healthy alternative to meat and potatoes. In fact, in the early 1970s it was reported that rats fed cardboard cereal boxes mixed with sugar, milk, and raisins fared better than those fed the cereal itself.[9, 10] Whether it was healthful or not (certainly the value of extreme fortification has been and is still questioned), this negative press sparked a fortification movement in the 1970s.

Nutrition According to Nineteenth-Century Science and Uncle Sam

Wilbur O. Atwater, a notable nutritionist in his time and the first director of nutritional research at the U.S. Department of Agriculture, wrote several articles in the late 1880s for *Century Magazine* about dietary issues. In these articles he endorsed the concept of decreasing meat and sugar intake. However, the reasons why he felt that meat consumption should be reduced primarily involved economics, conservation, and lastly health issues. He recognized the importance of the nutrients in meat for health but high quality meat was expensive, thus, Atwater suggested that Americans should substitute less expensive foods for meat. Certain foods supply the necessary nutrients of meat but can be obtained less expensively than meat. Beans and oatmeal are good sources of protein; these should often be substituted for expensive meat, and margarine could be used in place of butter (as one might expect, the dairy industry protested this). According to Atwater many poor and working-class people devoted too much of their income to food and, thus, they inefficiently used the little money that they had available on high-quality meat products. In those days it was a status symbol to be able to purchase high-quality meat for your family even if it left little money for other necessities of life.[11, 12] Other authors have also indicated that meat products were a symbol of pride and prosperity to the common people in this country 100 years ago.[13] Atwater was writing before vitamins had been discovered, according to today's standards of nutrition Atwater's recommendations would likely have promoted malnutrition rather than good health. For example, Atwater advised the poor to eat more white bread because it was inexpensive and fewer potatoes. Further, according to Atwater green vegetables, if consumed at all, should only be eaten when cooked in order to be digested easily.[14]

Additionally, Atwater noted repeatedly that Americans were particularly wasteful (compared to Europeans) when it came to food (too much was thrown away). Atwater was a conservationist: he believed that Americans worked harder and were more intelligent than Europeans and he attributed these qualities primarily to the land, or more precisely, the foods that came from the American soil. To him, the soil in America was richer in nutrients than the over-cultivated and depleted soil found in Europe: this fact allowed the United States to produce more high-quality food and in greater abundance than what was possible in European countries. He considered raising animals for food a less efficient method to produce protein and more destructive to the soil than growing certain high-protein crops.[11, 12, 15] A similar sentiment was raised a century later by Frances Lappe who authored *Diet for a Small Planet* (1971)[16] and is popular today among those who favor vegetarianism. The idea that soil depletion reduces the nutrients available in the vegetation grown in it is a concept that has been used frequently by vitamin-supplement dealers over the years. However, this generally has been characterized as a myth (i.e., the chemical composition of soil has no or very little effect on the vitamin content of products grown in it).[17-19]

Regarding the health value of meat and the nutrients found in meat, Atwater generally did not condemn or vilify dietary fat. He recognized it was a good source of energy for very active people and particularly those living in cold climates. However, for sedentary people and those who spent most of their time indoors it would be healthful to reduce fat intake as well as food consumption in general.[12] From all accounts it appears that experts (including Atwater) in the late nineteenth century considered many Americans to be gluttons. Accordingly, in the late 1800s several products became available to deal with our discomforts (i.e., patent medicines), including those associated with overeating (then referred to as dyspepsia and now as indigestion). Many of these "healthful" products contained ingredients like cocaine, alcohol, opiates, and marijuana, and some were the ancestors of our modern-day soft drinks. Coca-Cola, which initially contained both cocaine and caffeine, became available in this period and was endorsed as being a generally healthful (if not medicinal) beverage. Atwater also seemed to echo some of the views described by vegetarians like Graham and Kellogg: he considered certain ingredients in animal flesh to have stimulant properties—according to him like "caffeine" and "alcohol." Atwater indicated that eating animal flesh makes dogs "fierce" and "invigorates" people.[15]

Digesting this Early Work

The general notion among all of these early nutrition experts was that "you are what you eat, " thus, eating animals would give us animal-like characteristics. This sentiment was very evident among the counterculture enthusiasts of the late 1960s and according to Paul Rozin this attitude is still operating in our culture (particularly among the most educated) and causes a dilemma, we distinguish ourselves from animals but we become more like animals by eating them.[20] Perhaps this philosophy is in part responsible for the negative reputation (in terms of healthfulness) toward animal products and components of animal products that is so evident today. If so, nowadays, the emphasis has changed from the original idea that eating meat causes dyspepsia, sex, and aggression to the idea that eating meat (or at least the fat in meat) causes us to become fat and causes fatty deposits in blood vessels. The notion that "you are what you eat" is evident in both the earlier and modern viewpoints. Many people including some "experts" still believe that "we only get fat by eating fat."[21] Although this actually was once a controversy, we have known for over 150 years that the body does make fat from the carbohydrates and protein that are consumed.[22] A controversy apparently remains concerning the extent to which carbohydrates and protein contribute to obesity.

One of the more rewarding aspects of researching this book involved examining information about nutritional thinking from the nineteenth and early twentieth centuries. Some authors on the subject of nutrition have provided some interesting if not bizarre information. For example, C. C. Furnas and S. M. Furnas of Yale University and the University of Minnesota respectively (both prestigious institutions) wrote back in the 1930s about the tastiness and healthfulness of human flesh and how it is recommended for those with "delicate stomachs." The notion apparently being that they considered it most healthful for humans to eat things most like themselves because the body could process this material more quickly and easily. How they became so adamant about the tastiness of human flesh is a mystery.[23]

In spite of the reference to the health benefits of consuming human flesh, there are many similarities between the health reputation of foods today and the status of those same foods (in terms of wholesomeness) in the distant past (before the advent of vitamins). Comparisons of past versus present reputations for specific foods (e.g., potatoes) will be discussed in much greater detail in chapter six. Thus, a major determinant of a food reputation today is often that same food's reputation a century ago. There is an obvious parallel here with drug reputations, which also have their roots in the nineteenth and early twentieth centuries. College students believe certain types of drugs to be much more harmful to health than other types of drugs. For example, cocaine has a very negative reputation and has limited medical use in the United States (it is used legally as a surgical anesthetic). Drugs derived from opium (e.g., morphine and heroin) also have an extremely negative reputation and heroin has no legitimate medical use in the United States today.[24] Both cocaine and the opiate drugs were considered the miracle drugs of their day, so how did they acquire their negative image? The origins of their unsavory reputations certainly go back to the late nineteenth and early twentieth centuries and as with food reputations, to some extent, are impacted by social as much as scientific factors. Many people familiar with drug history in the United States have indicated that racism played a prominent role in American views (and ultimately the legal restrictions) concerning these drugs. Opium was associated to a large extent in the nineteenth century with Chinese laborers and cocaine with black Americans. Marijuana, which by the way does not have a particularly bad reputation in terms of health among college students today, was originally connected to Mexicans and black musicians. Thus, whether or not these drugs deserve their current reputations concerning health is open to debate, however, it is widely accepted that the roots of their reputations go back a century or more and, in part, are based in racial bias.[25]

Welcome to the Jungle

One event or series of events that appropriately influenced the reputation of meat in the early twentieth century was the publication of Upton Sinclair's novel, *The Jungle*, in February 1906. Sinclair was a socialist who was interested in improving working conditions. He was disappointed upon discovering that the readers of his book were more interested in the safety of the meat supply than the horrible labor conditions in the packing plants in Chicago. Although Sinclair's book was fiction his publisher investigated the issue and substantiated his depiction of meat processing immediately after he submitted the book for publication. The publisher (Doubleday) went on to publish magazine articles which contained additional facts, even worse than what Sinclair had first described, about the methods used in meat processing (e.g., diseased animals were being butchered for meat). President Theodore Roosevelt received copies of these articles and organized his own committee who investigated and ultimately confirmed that butchering practices were indeed terrible Meanwhile, Sinclair was publishing newspaper articles telling things that he had left out of his book. The press acquired and published all of these papers, even the report from the committee appointed by the president and a public furor ensued concerning this issue that swept the country. There was little opposition to this indignation for a few months later (June 30, 1906) the president signed the Meat Inspection Law and it went into effect the very next day.[26] Aside from meat, there were more general concerns about food processors' use of dangerous food additives and adulterants at this time, and these concerns led to the Pure Food and Drugs Act which was also passed in 1906.

Food Frets in the Great Depression

Although many people played important roles in the discovery of vitamins, Casimir Funk, who was looking for the anti-beriberi ingredient in rice hulls in 1912, is often given credit for this discovery. Funk went on to hypothesize that the diseases scurvy, beriberi, and pellagra were due to inadequate intakes of "vitamins:"[27] before this time it was commonly assumed that what we now know as vitamin deficiency diseases were caused by infections or toxins. Soon after the discovery of vitamins and the realization that diseases can be caused by their deficiencies many people became concerned that modern food processing (primarily milling and canning) was robbing foods of their essential nutrients. White flour, in spite of the early warnings by Graham, generally had a wholesome reputation until this time. However, although the large food processors made every attempt to assure the public that white bread was healthful (e.g., they enlisted the help of the American Medical Association and notable nutritionists), many people were skeptical and rightfully so.[28] This was before white flour was enriched and white flour without enrichment offers very little in terms of vitamins and minerals. Eventually this concern led to fortification of many commercial products with synthetic vitamins, however, the food industry was not eager to fortify their products at first for fear that it would be an admission that their products were lacking to begin with. The technology for synthetic production of vitamins came in the mid 1930s and quickly sparked the vitamin supplement (i.e., vitamins in pill or liquid form) industry. The processors were ultimately pushed toward fortification only when technology became available to measure nutrients in foods and show that some types of processing did in fact lower nutrient levels in foods. The American Medical Association (AMA) originally recommended fortifying processed foods but only as a means to bring vitamin levels in processed foods back to their original natural levels. Food processors, however, were often more eager to add loads of additional vitamins to foods (more than they ever had to begin with) and even to candy (a good source for additional information on this subject is Levenstein, 1993).[29]

The fortification movement was given a shot in the arm when Mayo Clinic researches reported in 1940 that thiamine deficiency caused sluggishness, decreased morale, and fatigue. In fact, it was rumored that Hitler was implementing thiamine starvation in order to control the energy and morale of those in the countries subdued by his armies. Further, given that modern milling processes removed most of the thiamine when producing white flour, many nutrition experts in the United States feared that American citizens were thiamine deficient and that this condition would not be conducive to withstanding the demands and stressors of war[30]or perhaps even an invasion[31]should this occur (this was a bit before Pearl Harbor). Thus, beginning in February of 1941 the United States began producing white flour enriched with thiamine, iron, and niacin.[32] One federal government official actually referred to thiamine as "the oomph vitamin."[33] This was probably the origin of the myth that vitamin supplements (i.e., extra vitamins) produce pep and vigor, which is commonly held today by many Americans. In the early 1940s thiamine likely had the most positive reputation of all the known vitamins, at least in the eyes of the public. A recent survey revealed that vitamin C is now revered much more than any other single vitamin, at least by grocery shoppers in northeast Pennsylvania. In fact, Americans possess many ideas regarding the benefits of vitamin supplement use that are not scientifically established. Americans (usually in excess of 90 percent of us) believe that even when our diet is adequate vitamin supplements can prevent or shorten illness, give extra strength or energy, prolong life, enhance memory and thinking, and help the body function better.[34]

Another food concern of the 1930s involved the presence of dangerous chemicals in commercial foods. Arsenic and lead compounds were sprayed on fruits to inhibit pests, while other potentially dangerous chemicals were used to make foods look fresh and preserve them.[35] According to food historian Harvey Levenstein these concerns ultimately did little more than spark sales of additive- and pesticide-free foods in health food stores and resulted in no significant legislation. The food industry was just too powerful and influential.[36]

Food Scares of the 1950s and 60s

Several events occurring in the late 1950s and early 1960s captured the public's attention and led to renewed fears about disease-causing chemicals in our food supply. Hormones fed to livestock, the presence of possible cancer-causing chemicals in foods, and perhaps most importantly the help of an aging movie star and health food enthusiast (i.e., Gloria Swanson) sparked the passage of legislation that forced processors to prove their food additives were safe. Determining food safety, in part, meant showing that the chemicals used in food processing did not promote disease in rodents.[37] A short time later on Thanksgiving of 1959 traces of a reported cancer-causing herbicide were found on cranberries.[38] The offensive berries were quickly removed from store shelves but shortly thereafter cancer-causing (at least in rats) poultry hormones and food colorings were discovered.[39] Further, if that was not enough the publication of a disquieting book entitled *Silent Spring* which foreboded massive extinction of many species (hence the word silent in the title because song birds were wiped out)[40] as a result of the use of chemical sprays and food additives assisted to awaken the slumbering consumer movement. Even the federal government admitted that trace amounts of the popular pesticide DDT were present in many of our foods and that this chemical tends to collect in fat tissue.[41] However it wasn't until 1962 when insight was provided by Rachel Carson (the author of *Silent Spring*) that this chemical also accumulates in human fat. The chemical companies and agribusiness countered successfully (at least for a while) by questioning Carson's expertise on the subject. But, Carson ultimately gained the upper hand and more credibility a few years later when it was reported that fish in the Great Lakes contained levels of mercury that were deadly to humans.[42] Sadly, although Rachel Carson is often credited for jumpstarting the environmental movement and her writing was likely instrumental to the eventual formation of the U.S. Environmental Protection Agency, she died in 1964, just two years after the publication of her alarming and eye-opening book.[43] The information concerning deadly mercury in our food supply caused more folks to accept Carson's earlier warnings.[42] "Organic" food producers and sellers were among the first to profit from this information. Even the nutrient value of non-organically produced foods was called into question by "organic" and "natural" advocates. Ultimately the large food processing companies were enlightened that the term "natural" (and more recently "fresh") on food labels was a natural gold mine and if anything directed the message toward women.[44] For example, starting in the early 1970s advertisers were churning up warm feelings of our more wholesome, natural, and rustic past with the introduction of granola under brand names like Heartland Nature Cereal, Nature Valley, and Country Morning. And, at this time the elderly Euell Gibbons, author of a best-selling guidebook on edible plants, revived enthusiasm for the natural and time-honored Grape Nuts.[7] Advertisers are still attempting to elicit feelings of bucolic nostalgia in cereal commercials. Kellogg is now (i.e., spring 2003) using the theme from *The Waltons* when advertising its new cereal Fruit Harvest.

As occurred in the 1930s food processing became a major issue: the revived notion that food processing rids foods of their nutrient contents became popular once again. In fact, the average person who didn't have the time and money for fancy health food regimens responded by taking more vitamins, sometimes in mega doses. This led to even more claims about the value of vitamin supplements, for example massive amounts of vitamin E were thought to prevent hair loss and vitamin C could cure the common cold. The AMA tried to stem this vitamin enthusiasm by alerting Americans to possible dangers of excessive vitamin consumption.[45] The FDA proclaimed that vitamin supplements were a waste of money because over-processing and soil depletion were myths: the FDA even advocated labels on vitamin packages indicating that vitamin supplements are not necessary. Congressional lobbyists for the powerful drug companies who made vitamin supplements squashed this movement by the FDA: congress even went a step further by severely limiting the FDA's power over vitamin sales.[46] In fact, although they were motivated by legitimate concerns about vitamin toxicity, the FDA has been halted on several occasions when attempting to regulate over-the-counter vitamins and vitamin-enriched foods like breakfast cereals. With the FDA crippled by congressional subjugation, fortification of ready-to-eat cereal soared (e.g., 14 percent of cereals were fortified in 1969 versus 92 percent in 1976).[27] The FDA's power to regulate so called "dietary supplements" is extremely limited, for example, supplement manufacturers are not required to provide evidence that their products are safe or effective before marketing them.[47]

Americans always hear that canned foods are nutritionally deficient at least compared to their raw or even their frozen counterparts. Upon researching this mainstream wisdom by comparing specific vitamin and mineral values for canned versus raw or frozen fruits and vegetables using *Bowes and Church's Food Values of Portions Commonly Used* by Jean Pennington[48] it became evident that this is sometimes not the case. Raw or frozen fruits and vegetables often had slightly more vitamins and minerals than an identical amount of the same product canned. However, the differences were almost always small and surprisingly sometimes the canned products had more vitamins and minerals than the raw version (e.g., for the foods pineapple and onions). Although sodium is an essential mineral for human life, due to its negative reputation, it was not included in these comparisons. Thus, the notion that canned foods have had all or most of their vitamins and minerals processed out of them seems to be an overstatement. As often publicized, the sodium levels were usually higher in the canned products and this was often most evident in canned vegetables rather than fruits.

In the 1960s and early 1970s activists like Ralph Nader and others who were disenchanted with government and big business applied significant pressure on food processors. For example, the practices of meat-packing houses were called into question once again (hotdogs were considered by some to be composed of little more than fat and rodent hair).[49] Additionally, many products (e.g., even baby foods) were reported to be produced and processed with excessive amounts of fat, sugar, sodium, untested additives, pesticides, hormones, and antibiotics. Further, the food manufacturers even attacked one another, for example, the sugar industry financed research to besmear non-caloric sweeteners and the makers of non-caloric sweeteners investigated the dangers of sugar. Finally, although some had been reporting relationships between blood cholesterol and disease for many years few people considered the issue worthy of their concern until it was reported in the late 1950s that polyunsaturated fats may lower blood cholesterol levels. Food makers who manufactured products that contained polyunsaturated fats (e.g., margarine, salad dressing) could not pass up the opportunity to disseminate information concerning their products' reported health benefits to the public.[50] Thus, food manufacturers provided what some would consider to be half-baked scientific information to the public that resulted in the beginning of the cholesterol and saturated fat concern and a decline in the consumption of traditionally wholesome products like dairy products. It took a few years but the United States government ultimately gave credence to the anti-cholesterol and anti-fat movement particularly as they pertain to diseases of the heart.

Food issues of the 1980s and 90s

In the later part of the 1980s a fervor did arise over the use of a pesticide and growth regulator with the trade name Alar. The chemical was used primarily on apples and in 1989 it suddenly became implicated as a carcinogenic agent with a fondness for small children (mostly because kids eat lots of apple products). It ultimately became known that only about 10 to 20 percent of apples were treated with Alar and that raw apples were never a threat because Alar itself was actually not the offensive agent. Instead a breakdown product of Alar that was produced only by exposing Alar to intense heat during the processing of apple juice was the culprit. Although the maker of Alar provided research suggesting that Alar was not hazardous given that a hungry baby did not consume more than 19, 000 quarts of apple juice daily, they did pull the chemical off the market.[51] However, at least one author of a book printed in the year 2000 is still warning readers of the dangers of Alar in both raw apples and apple juice.[52]

A report from the American Medical Association provided a controversial perspective regarding pesticide risk. Most of us are concerned about synthetic pesticide residue in our foods, however, plants produce their own natural pesticides, particularly when stressed by invading insects, and many of these natural pesticides are known carcinogens. The report went on to say that these natural pesticides are much more abundant in foods (more than 15, 000 fold) than synthetic pesticides and more of the natural ones are carcinogenic. Thus, failure to use synthetic pesticides, it was argued, can substantially increase the amounts of cancer-causing chemicals in foods.[53]

The safety of beef consumption became a greater concern throughout the 1980s and 90s with the increased notoriety of Escherichia coli 0157:H7 (E. coli) and bovine spongiform encephalopathy (i.e., mad cow disease). Mad cow disease was identified in

1986 after it began striking cows in Great Britain, causing them to become uncoordinated and timid. The concern resulted in a worldwide ban on British beef and livestock imports and the slaughter and incineration of thousands of cattle in Great Britain. Although no one is certain about the identity of the disease-causing agent, one leading theory is that an aberrant protein (i.e., a prion) is to blame. The fear was (and still is) that the disease can be transmitted from animals to humans possibly from exposure to affected animals or consumption of contaminated meat.[54, 55] E. coli was categorized as a human pathogen by the Centers for Disease Control in 1982. It is a variant of a normal gut bacteria which can live in the intestines of healthy animals, however, meat can become contaminated during slaughter. Affected meat must be adequately cooked, rare meat consumption is the primary method of transmission in humans. The infection can produce gastrointestinal illness and occasionally kidney failure and death.[56] Many cases of E coli in the United States have been linked to ground beef purchased at fast food restaurants.[57, 58] To what extent concerns such as this (rather than dietary fat) influence people to avoid beef products is unknown. However, when asked to rate hamburgers or Big Macs in terms of healthfulness respondents report concerns about fat and never mention E coli or mad cow disease.[59-63] Certainly, the average American is eating less red meat compared to twenty years ago. Further, Time magazine recently reported that vegetarianism is in fashion and that most people cite health rather than the taste of meat or concern for animals as their primary reason.[64]

A reportedly healthful component of the grain seed known as bran was injected into the public consciousness like never before in the mid 1980s by the cereal industry. Bran is the outside portion of the grain seed, it does not dissolve in water and is often referred to as fiber or roughage. With white flour the bran, along with its accompanying vitamins, are removed. The Kellogg Company launched the bran craze with television ads describing high-bran diets as cancer inhibitors. It wasn't long before reduction of heart disease was included as a benefit with much of the health-promoting publicity associated with eating oat bran. No interference came from the federal government, at least not initially, in fact the bran campaign was praised by the Federal Trade Commission. By 1989 store shelves were invaded with products like oat bran donuts, milkshakes, waffles, pasta, pretzels, potato chips, and even oat bran beer. The government (at both the federal and state levels) ultimately became concerned about the unsubstantiated health claims or what one reporter called "bran washing." The Nutrition Labeling and Education Act, negative media attention, and a bit of scientific dissent concerning bran's cholesterol's reducing qualities eventually cooled the bran hysteria.[65]

Summary and Conclusions

A description of the more major social events and people in the history of America that have influenced food reputations was provided in this chapter. Concerns about meat products extend back to the early nineteenth century with the preaching of William Sylvester Graham. Meat trepidation has reached a zenith in the past few decades with the mistrust of processed meats and campaigns against dietary fat and cholesterol. Some of this concern regarding meat products throughout American history may be influenced by the enduring conviction that "we are what we eat." The reputations of diary products and eggs have suffered for similar reasons but probably to a lesser extent. A primary aim of this chapter was to provide an explanation as to how food characteristics such as freshness, natural, and unprocessed have become important to Americans. Recent surveys have indicated the importance of freshness to Americans.[66] For example, perhaps perceptions of characteristics such as freshness in foods may partially explain why food name and food description ratings are often not in agreement. That is, certain food names (e.g., apple) may connote freshness to Americans, while the nutrient description for the apple would not. Attempts were made in this chapter to describe rather than enhance or contribute to food reputations: the goal of this writing was not to arouse political sensitivities. Other writers have devoted their time and efforts to exploring the politics of nutrition, food, and eating in America.[13, 67, 68]

Notes

1. G. Carson, *Cornflake crusade* (New York: Rinehart and Company, Inc. 1957).
2. S. Bruce, and B. Crawford, *Cerealizing America: The unsweetened story of American breakfast cereal* (Boston: Faber and Faber 1995), p. 4.
3. Carson, *Cornflake crusade*, p. 34.
4. Carson, *Cornflake crusade*, p. 34.

5. Carson, *Cornflake crusade*, p. 35.
6. R. Crooks, and K. Baur, Our Sexuality (New York: The Benjamin/Cummings Publishing Company, Inc. 1993).
7. Bruce, and Crawford, *Cerealizing America*.
8. H. Levenstein, *Revolution at the table* (New York: Oxford University Press 1988). 22.
9. Bruce, and Crawford, *Cerealizing America*. 230.
10. J. Rosenthal, Hunger expert says many dry cereals are not nutritious, *New York Times* (Friday, July 24, 1970) 1.
11. W. O. Atwater, What we should eat, *Century Magazine* 36 (1888), 257-264.
12. W. O. Atwater, Pecuniary economy of food, *Century Magazine* 36 (1888), 257-264.
13. L. S. Sims, *The politics of fat* (Armonk, NY: M. E. Sharpe 1998).
14. W. O. Atwater, How food nourishes the body, *Century Magazine* 34 (1887) 237.
15. W. O. Atwater, The chemistry of food and nutrition, *Century Magazine* 36 (1887), 257-264.
16. F. M. Lappe, *Diet for a small planet*, (New York: Ballantine, 1975).
17. M. Castleman, The myth and promise of organic produce. *Medical Self-Care,* fall (1981).
18. L. B. Jensen, *Man's foods: Nutrition and environments in food gathering times and food producing times* (Champaign, IL: The Garrard Press 1953) 232.
19. 37. J. V. Young, *The medical messiahs: A social history of health quackery in twentieth-century America* (Princeton, NJ: Princeton University Press 1967), 351.
20. P. Rozin, Towards a psychology of food and eating: From motivation to module to model to marker, morality, meaning, and metaphor, *Current Directions in Psychological Science* 5 (1996), 18-24.
21. M. Nestle, R. Wing, L. Birch, L. DiSogra, et al. Behavioral and social influences on food choice, *Nutritional Reviews* 56 (1998), S50-S74.
22. E. V. McCollum, *A History of nutrition: The sequence of ideas in nutritional investigations* (Boston: Houghton Mifflin Company 1957) 36.
23. C. C. Furnas and S. M. Furnas, *Man, Bread and destiny*, (New York: Reynal and Hitchcock 1937).
24. M. E. Oakes, Beauty or beast: Stereotypes of familiar drugs, manuscript submitted to the *Journal of Drug Education.*
25. D. F. Musto, Opium, Cocaine, and Marijuana in American History, *Scientific American* (July, 1991) 40-47.
26. I. D. Garard, *The story of food* (Westport, CT: The AVI Publishing Company, Inc. 1974) 76-77.
27. J. Backstrand, The history and future of food fortification in the United States: A public health perspective, *Nutritional reviews* 60 (2002), 15-26.
28. F. J. Schlink, *Eat drink and be wary* (New York: Covici Friede Publishers 1935) 13-33.
29. H. Levenstein, *Paradox of plenty: A social history of eating in modern America* (New York: Oxford University Press 1993) 19-21.
30. R. M. Wilder, Hitler's secret weapon is depriving people of vitamin, *Science News Letter* (April 12, 1941).
31. No author, Vitamins for war, *Journal of the American Medical Association* 115 (Oct. 5, 1940) 1198-1199.
32. No author, Vitamin-enriched flour goes into production, *Science News Letter* (February 8, 1941) 83-84.

33. Federal Security Agency Office of the Director of Defense, Health and Welfare Services (1942). Proceedings of the national nutrition conference for defense (May 1941), 37.
34. M. E. Oakes, E. Corrigan, S. Alaimo, T. Bator, E. Vagner, C. S. Slotterback, Vitamin supplement myths (unpublished).
35. A. Kallet, and F. J. Schlink, 100, 000, 000 guinea pigs (New York: Grosset and Dunlap 1933) 47-60.
36. H. Levenstein, *Paradox of plenty: A social history of eating*, 17.
37. R. D. Lyons, Congressman says actress's speech helped bar cyclamates, *New York Times* (Wednesday, October 22, 1959) 26.
38. No author, How pure is your food? *U. S. News and World Report* (Dec. 7, 1959).
39. No author, Food additives arouse dispute, *New York Times* (Sunday, June 30, 1957) 34.
40. R. L. Carson, *Silent Spring* (Cambridge, MA: The Riverside Press 1962).
41. No author, Survey shows DDT is present in foods, *New York Times* (Saturday, October 16 1954) 19.
42. H. Levenstein, *Paradox of plenty: A social history of eating*, 162.
43. B. Watson, Sounding the Alarm, *Smithsonian* (September 2002) 115-117.
44. H. Levenstein, *Paradox of plenty: A social history of eating*, 108.
45. P. Bart, Food and drug businesses gird for war over use of vitamins, *New York Times* (Tuesday, April 25, 1961) 47.
46. H. Levenstein, *Paradox of plenty: A social history of eating*, 166-169.
47. A. Spake, Natural hazards, *U.S. News and World Report*. February 12, 2001, 43-49.
48. J. A. T. Pennington, *Bowes and Church's Food values of portions commonly used* (Philadelphia, PA: Lippincott 1998).
49. H. Wellford, *Sowing the Wind* (New York: Grossman Publishers 1972).
50. H. Levenstein, *Paradox of plenty: A social history of eating*, 170-176.
51. S. Gebo, *What's left to eat?* (New York: McGraw Hill, Inc. 1992) 6-7.
52. R. Yaron, *Super baby food* (Archibald, PA: F. J. Roberts Publishing Company 2000) 64 and 425.
53. Council on Scientific Affairs, Diet and cancer: where do we stand, *Archives of Internal Medicine* 153 (1993), 50-56.
54. S. B. Prusiner, The prion diseases, *Scientific American*, January, 1995, 48-57.
55. T. Beardsley, Deadly enigma, *Scientific American*, December, 1996, 16-18.
56. *http://www.cdc.gov/ncidod/dbmd/diseaseinfo/escherichiacoli_g.htm*
57. N. Fox, *Spoiled: The dangerous truth about a food chain gone haywire* (New York: Basic Books 1997).
58. E. Schlosser, *Fast food nation: the dark side of the all-American meal* (New York: Houghton Mifflin Company 2001).
59. M. E. Oakes and C. S. Slotterback, Gender differences in perceptions of the healthiness of foods, *Psychology and Health* 16 (2001[a]), 57-65.
60. M. E. Oakes and C. S. Slotterback, What's in a name? A comparison of men's and women's judgements about food names and their nutrient contents, *Appetite* 36 (2001[b]), 29-40.
61. M. E. Oakes and C. S. Slotterback, Judgements of food healthfulness: food name stereotypes in adults over age 25, *Appetite* 37 (2001[c]), 1-8.
62. M. E. Oakes, Differences in Judgments of Food Healthfulness by Young and Elderly Women, *Food Quality and Preference* 14 (2003) 227-236.
63. M. E. Oakes, An examination of the influence of gender and dieting status on ratings of food healthfulness. In S. P. Anderson, ed.: *Advances in psychology research 16* (New York: Nova Science Publishers 2002).

64. R. Corliss, Should we all be vegetarians? *Time* July 15, (2002), 48-56.

65. Bruce and Crawford, *Cerealizing America*. 235-240.

66. M. E. Oakes and C. S. Slotterback, The good, the bad, and the ugly: Characteristics used by young, middle-aged, and older men and women, dieters and non-dieters to judge the healthfulness of foods, *Appetite* 38 (2002), 91-97.

67. D. Maurer and J. Sobal, *Eating Agenda: Food and nutrition as social problems* (New York: Aldine De Gruyter 1995).

68. M. Nestle, *Food politics: How the food industry influences nutrition and health* (Berkeley: University of California Press 2002).

3

The Fat is in the Fire

An Introduction to Fat

Perhaps no other nutrition message in American history has influenced food reputations to the extent of the anti-fat campaign of the past few decades. Dietary fat content is the primary characteristic used by men when determining the healthfulness of foods and often the only characteristic used by women.[1, 2]

Although we rarely if ever hear this message from the popular press, fats are vitally important for human life for several reasons: (1) they are a major component of all of the cell membranes in our body; (2) they are a basic ingredient in the production of many hormones and other physiologically important substances; (3) they protect and insulate the organs of the body; (4) dietary fat aids in the absorption of fat-soluble vitamins (e.g., vitamins A, D, E, and K); (5) fat makes up a large portion of our nervous system including the brain and are essential for nervous system communication. In fact, multiple sclerosis is a progressive disease resulting in the destruction of the fatty tissue responsible for maintaining nervous system communication. Although this information is far from penetrating the public consciousness, as will soon be described, much of the recent research concerning dietary fat concerns its potential health benefits to many organ systems of the body (e.g., the heart and brain).

Fatty acids are components of fat and are paramount to our health. When animals are not allowed access to the important fatty acids (research that would clearly be unethical to pursue using human participants) they become emaciated, their heart enlarges, their immune system is sacrificed, and reproductive abilities are weakened. Many fatty acids can be made from the foods that we eat but two fatty acids can only be obtained through dietary sources and are thus referred to as essential fatty acids. There are many types of fatty acids and they can be classified as saturated or unsaturated depending on their chemical structure. The unsaturated fatty acids can be further divided into monounsaturated and polyunsaturated varieties. These facts are among the few that are not in question concerning dietary fat.

Cholesterol is a lipid that is found only in animal tissues. Although very important for our existence, it is not an essential component of our diets due to the fact that our bodies produce sufficient amounts to meet our needs. Contrary to what we usually hear from medical staff and media there are not "good" and "bad" types of cholesterol, only cholesterol itself. Lipoproteins (e.g., LDL and HDL) refer to large molecules that are responsible for carrying cholesterol around the body. The wisdom is that LDL molecules carry necessary cholesterol to our tissues for use. However, the hypothesis is that excessive depositing of cholesterol by LDL molecules can lead to narrowing of blood vessels. On the other hand, HDL molecules are thought to remove cholesterol from cells and transport it back to the liver where it can be excreted.[3, 4] The term "cholesterol profile" will be used to refer to a ratio of LDL and HDL in this chapter.

Be Cautious about Dietary Fat Research

One of the first sources encountered when investigating food reputations for this chapter was the book *Nutritional Epidemiology* written by Harvard's Walter Willett, a most notable figure in nutrition research. As expected, Willett indicated that knowing the absolute amounts of certain nutrients (e.g., total calories) consumed by individuals does allow a researcher to predict to some degree who will develop coronary heart disease in the future. However, it was stunning to discover that people who consume more calories are less likely to develop coronary heart disease. Further, knowing a person's consumption in grams of total dietary fat, saturated fat, and cholesterol is not predictive of whether the person will develop heart disease, in fact, if anything those who remain healthy may consume slightly more of these nutrients. How can this be? Well, the most widely accepted explanation used to account for this phenomena is that physically active people tend to eat more, thus, they consume more calories than sedentary people. As a result physically active people generally consume more of most nutrients even those with negative reputations. Thus, the fact that people who take in higher amount of calories are more likely to remain heart disease free is thought to be a testimony to the benefits of exercise.[5]

The message just stated hopefully sounds reasonable but the reader is still likely wondering how this can be true given the enormity and intensity of the negative messages about the supposed sinister nutrient dietary fat. The logic goes like this: those of us who are very inactive may eat a bit less than those of us who are very active, but inactive people consume a higher percentage of their total calories from dietary fat. Thus, it is the percentage of total calories from dietary fat (and not total grams of dietary fat) that has been shown in some studies to be predictive of heart disease. However, it would be deceptive if one neglected to mention that some studies have found no relationship between percentage of calories from dietary fat (or even saturated fat) and heart disease.[5]

Further, it is important to understand that when one thing (e.g., percentage of saturated fat) predicts another (e.g., heart disease) or when two events (or in this case measures) are said to be correlated or associated we have a powerful tendency to believe that one is causing the other: this is a mistake. To illustrate, the number of people wearing gloves (one measure) and the number of people having chapped lips (a second measure) are correlated or associated. But, this does not mean that wearing gloves causes chapped lips or that having chapped lips causes us to wear gloves. Climatic conditions (a third measure) cause both chapped lips and glove wearing. Similarly, in 1990, when the low-fat craze was approaching high gear, Walter Willett related "it is ironic that the existing studies of diet and coronary heart disease provide better support for the influence of exercise than they do for any primary effect of diet."[6] Perhaps astonishing to many readers, the dietary factor that has been most consistently correlated with heart health over the past few decades is alcohol consumption. Consumption of one or two drinks each day of wine, beer, or liquor is associated with reduced risk of coronary heart disease.[7] However, as I tell my students, there is no evidence that abstaining until Saturday night then binging to catch up is healthful.

The Reputation of Fatty Acids

In the consciousness of most lay people all types of dietary fat are both unhealthful and promoters of obesity. It is true that all types of fat are identical concerning their caloric content and that dietary fat has over twice as many calories (nine calories per gram) than either carbohydrates or protein (both having about four calories per gram). However, saturated fatty acids have a particularly negative reputation among both lay people and the scientific community for contributing to diseases of the heart and obesity, and to a lesser extent cancer. There are four saturated fatty acids that are abundant in both animal and vegetable fats, three of which (i.e., lauric acid, myristic acid, and palmitic acid) are viewed as unhealthful by most nutritional researchers particularly concerning their reported effects on the heart. The other abundant saturated fatty acid (stearic acid) generally has a neutral reputation concerning health (e.g., not helping or harming the heart). Due to its harmless reputation, some people are advocating the exclusion of stearic acid (which is abundant in chocolate) from the saturated fatty acid tally on food labels.[8]

The monounsaturated fatty acids (e.g., oleic acid) have been in high favor among some nutrition researchers for several years now but are not viewed as positively by most lay people. A great deal of research attention has been devoted to investigating something called the Mediterranean diet. Those who live in countries that surround the Mediterranean (Crete gets mentioned a lot) have been reported to have a low incidence of coronary heart disease and some types of cancer (e.g., breast and prostate cancer). Some scientists attribute these reported health advantages to the high consumption of olive oil by the inhabitants of this region. Olive oil has an abundance of oleic acid (i.e., a monounsaturated fatty acid) and has also been reported to promote a healthy blood lipid (e.g., cholesterol) profile and be helpful to those with diabetes. Scientists are currently crowing over this nutrient to the extent that some have boldly stated that there is no reason to restrict this nutrient in our diets unless perhaps obesity is a major concern.[9] In addition to olive oil, major sources of monounsaturated fat include canola oils, nuts, and avocados.

Polyunsaturated fatty acids are also viewed positively by a sizeable portion of the scientific community and a few health-conscious lay people. The two essential dietary fatty acids for humans are both of the polyunsaturated type and are referred to as linoleic acid and linolenic acids. Polyunsaturated fats like linolenic acid, which is abundant in many vegetable oils (particularly flaxseed oil), and the fatty acids found in the flesh of certain marine animals (e.g., salmon and sardines) currently have the blessing of many dietary-fat researchers. These marine fats as well as linolenic acid are often together referred to as omega-3 fatty acids and are being highly (but not universally) touted these days for their healthful effects on the heart mostly but also the bones, nervous system, and for cancer prevention. Interestingly, it was noticed almost 150 years ago that Eskimos living in Greenland tended to bleed for extended periods of time (their blood takes longer to clot when injured). This ineffi-ciency concerning blood clotting may be advantageous in terms of heart disease. The hypothesis is that eating lots of fish and fish-eating mammals may inhibit blood clotting and as a consequence decrease heart fatalities.[10] Marine animal fat is not essential in our diets, in fact, our bodies can make their own marine fatty acids out of linolenic acid. The scientists who are raving about omega-3 fatty acids claim that they reduce our risk of sudden cardiac death, i.e., when people die within minutes because their heart stops beating. Omega-3 fatty acids are thought to stabilize the heart's electrical activity and, thus, make the heart more resistant to these poten-tially fatal events. Additionally, omega-3 fatty acids have been re-ported to have favorable effects on blood lipids (e.g., cholesterol) and make blood clotting less likely. Further, the benefits of the vaunted Mediterranean diet that was described earlier are now be-ing attributed to omega-3 fatty acid consumption as much (if not more) than olive oil. Those Mediterranean folks are thought to be extremely fortunate, it has been reported that even the average Greek chicken egg has ten times more omega-3 fatty acids than do our chicken eggs.[11] Interestingly, some of the recent studies investigat-ing the healthful effects of omega-3 fatty acid consumption found reductions in likelihood of dieing but no changes in serum choles-terol, suggesting that blood cholesterol may not be the consum-mate measure of heart disease risk as it has so often been promoted.[12] This information concerning the health benefits of dietary fat has prompted the American Heart Association to recommend at least two servings of fish per week and has caused some investigators to question the widespread use of fat-free foods such as salad dress-ing and mayonnaise.[13]

Deficiencies in essential fatty acids are rare in adults but have been observed in children fed extremely low-fat diets: skin abnormalities are the most prominent symptoms of severe fat restriction in children.[3] Some parents have become so swept up in the fat hysteria that they place their infants or young children on low-fat diets with unhealthful results such as this as the consequence.[14] Mainstream pediatric physicians emphasize the extreme importance of dietary fats for babies and young children for growth and nervous system development.

Although popular in the American diet, not all unsaturated fatty acids have a healthful reputation among nutritional scientists. Trans-fatty acids are unsaturated and found naturally in some foods (e.g., milk fat) but most are produced in the process of making margarine, shortening, and frying oils. Thus, trans-fatty acids are common in baked goods and fried foods.[3] Trans-fatty acids are reputed to alter blood cholesterol profiles in an unfavorable manner and as a consequence, according to some researchers, may promote blood clotting and consequently heart disease and strokes. Some authorities have also suggested that trans-fatty acids may contribute to diabetes.[13] Other authorities (a minority) warn that the jury is still out regarding the dangers of trans-fatty acids and that their vilification may be unjustified.[9]

From Pork to Nuts

Does pork really deserve its negative reputation? Pork was the most commonly consumed meat throughout most of American history (overtaken by beef in 1955). In the nineteenth century (i.e., before refrigeration) pork was typically preserved using salt, that is, typically in the form of hams and sausage. In fact, hogs and hominy were mainstay fare throughout much of America in the nineteenth century.[15] Although pork was consumed frequently by the middle class, they along with the upper class viewed pork quite negatively in terms of healthfulness: it was considered extremely unwholesome, and difficult to digest (i.e., it was thought to cause dyspepsia).[16] More recently, seventy years ago, many Americans believed that pork consumption increased sexual passion and the image of pork, if anything, has deteriorated since then.[17] Of course like many animal products, pork has a negative reputation in terms of healthfulness these days in the United States due to a large extent to the exorbitant levels of fat that have been reported in pork products. However, the reader may be surprised to discovered that almost 50 percent of the fatty acid content in a pork chop is monounsaturated fat, most of it being oleic acid which is also abundant in olive oil and has received a great deal of positive press over the years concerning its benefits to the heart. About 12 percent of the fatty acids in a pork chop are polyunsaturated fat the most abundant being linoleic acid, which is an essential fatty acid and has also been praised for its health benefits. The rest (38 percent) is saturated fat but a third of that is stearic acid, which is not considered a health hazard by most nutritional scientists. Thus, almost two-thirds of the fat in a pork chop has a positive reputation for healthfulness among many scientists, 13 percent is neutral in terms of healthfulness, and the rest, about 25 percent, is considered to be harmful.[18] Additionally, a fried pork chop has about 28 percent of the recommended daily value of cholesterol, in contrast, one egg has just over 70 percent of the recommended value for cholesterol.[19] However, nutritional scientists are often giving eggs a thumbs-up in part because dietary cholesterol is now thought to have a minimal impact on both blood cholesterol and coronary heart disease for most of us. Just on the basis of this information one could argue that pork does not deserve its unwholesome reputation in the lay and scientific communities.

Even the type of fat in the much-maligned Big Mac, which seems to hold the dubious distinction as being the king of junk fare in the United States, is mostly (i.e., 68 percent) unsaturated. And, about one third of the saturated fat is the reputed harmless (in terms of heart health) stearic acid. The remarkable abundance and variety of vitamins and minerals in the Big Mac have already been described.

No one except possibly those associated with pork production or McDonald's are promoting pork and Big Macs as being healthful. However, some fatty foods tend to have a negative reputation in the lay world but are currently in favor with many nutritional scientists. Nuts are a good example of foods that are traditionally avoided in the United States because of their fat content (e.g., 86 percent of the energy in walnuts comes from fat). The reputation of nuts among fat researchers is anything but ominous, nut consumption has been associated with reduced heart disease risks and an improved cholesterol profile.[13] Although several types of nuts have been lauded by scientists (e.g., peanuts and almonds) walnuts have received some of the best publicity in the scientific literature, black walnuts are very high in polyunsaturated fatty acids, have moderate amounts of monounsaturated fat, and a little saturated fat.[19] Recently it was observed that some walnut packages now have "omega 3" printed in large letters on the front panel of their labels but the words "fat or fatty" were left out.

How did Dietary Fat Become so Vilified?

Although some scientists claim that the role of dietary lipids in causing heart disease is well established,[20] it is now recognized by some of the most prominent dietary-fat researchers in the world that the low-fat campaign is based on scant scientific evidence and that the half-baked nutritional messages that caused the vilification of all dietary fats likely resulted in unintended harm.[13] Thus, if dietary fat is so important for human life and if many types of dietary fat are considered beneficial to health according to a significant portion of the scientific community, why is this nutrient so demonized in the popular press and viewed as toxic by many Americans?

As stated in a previous chapter the origins of the reputation of meat as a primary scourge of human health and longevity can be attributed to the preachings of William Sylvester Graham. However, the introduction of scientific information to the tenant that dietary fat causes health problems began early in the twentieth century when it was observed that dietary fat consumption and levels of fatty deposits in blood vessels (often called atherosclerosis) were correlated in natives from Java and Dutch settlers living in the region. Other investigators were showing at about the same time that feeding rabbits extremely high-fat diets increased atherosclerosis.[21] This information did not attract widespread attention because at that time the masses were more concerned about under-nutrition than over-nutrition (sometimes called affluent malnutrition or negative nutrition). However, just after World War II a clamor arose about what seemed to many to be a dramatic increase in prevalence of coronary heart disease.

Many authors have indicated that heart disease was almost unheard of at the beginning of the twentieth century. Those who were writing at that time (e.g., Wilbur Atwater) made no mention of this disease, at least in the literature that was evaluated for this book.

Further, the first official recognition of the disease did not come until 1929 with the revised publication of the *International Lists of Diseases and Causes of Death.*[22] However, even though heart disease was considered rare the life expectancy at birth in 1900 was forty-six years compared to seventy-six years today. The leading causes of death in 1900 were related to infectious disease (e.g., pneumonia) and diarrheal diseases related to poor sanitation and malnutrition. Many authorities have attributed the reported increased incidence of heart disease that occurred in the mid-twentieth century to dietary changes. Although dietary changes may well account for some of the increase in the diagnosis of heart disease other non-dietary factors are also likely important, further, some of these non-dietary factors may not be particularly ominous. First, given that heart disease usually does not become life threatening until a person is either middle-aged or elderly, the mere fact that people are living longer would account for some of the increases that were reported. Second, since mortality rates for the primary killers of 100 years ago have fallen dramatically, diseases that were rare a century ago get more attention now. Third, heart disease even as a cause of death may have often gone unrecognized 100 years ago. The diagnostic category "diseases of the heart" was officially changed in 1949 to include a wider variety of diseases.[23] Further, there clearly was less certainty about the causes of death several decades ago, for example, it was not uncommon for acute indigestion to be mentioned as the cause of death on death certificates.[24] On a related note, better medical technology allows us to diagnose illnesses earlier and the advent and initial use of this technology would cause the number of diagnosed cases to increase temporarily.

In spite of these more optimistic interpretations of heart disease prevalence, dietary fat and cholesterol were suspected by some authorities to be the culprit in what some described as an epidemic rise in coronary heart disease. The uproar stimulated research interests dedicated to exploring relationships between diet and heart disease. Two of the most famous studies generated from this concern are known in the scientific literature as the Framingham Study and the Seven Countries Study (it was this study that sparked interest in the Mediterranean diet). These studies were among the first to establish a relationship between blood cholesterol and disease risk. The Seven Countries Study under the direction of Ancel Keys ultimately provided the most influential correlational data showing a relationship between consumption of saturated fat as a percentage of total calories and coronary heart disease. Basically it was reported that countries (e.g., Greece) consuming little saturated fat tended to have a lower incidence of coronary heart disease compared to, for example, Eastern Finland where people ate lots of saturated fat and held the dubious distinction of having the world's highest coronary rate.[25, 26] However, critics have always argued that other factors, for example, fruit and vegetable consumption or just plain overeating may account for this relationship. The early work (and warnings) from Keys concerning heart disease, which began in the mid-1940s, along with scant amounts of research relating dietary factors to blood cholesterol provoked organizations like the American Heart Associations to intensify their anticholesterol campaign by advising Americans to cut back on meat consumption. The ambiguity of the message about dietary fat and cholesterol as killers and the polarization of the scientific community on this subject allowed the federal government to mostly stay out of the fray and continue promoting the importance of the Basic Four Foods which many of us remember from elementary school. What broke the gridlock among scientists and ultimately directed the country toward the anti-fat campaign, of which we are all familiar, was not noteworthy scientific discoveries but instead the crusading of politicians. The Senate Select Committee on Nutrition and Human Needs was established in 1968 with Senator George McGovern as chairperson. The committee originally devoted its efforts to eradicating malnutrition in the United States, a notion that was politically popular in the late 1960s. However, in the early 1970s after McGovern's resounding defeat in the presidential election and when malnutrition became less politically hot the committee shifted its attention to the overfeeding of Americans. The fat ultimately went into the fire in February of 1977 when the committee issued the first edition of Dietary Goals for the United States.[23] This report was described as "revolutionary" which is probably appropriate given the controversy it provoked (even the American Medical Association opposed it) and the dramatic shift in position from previous government recommendations. For the first time we were being told by our government to eat less fat, cholesterol, sugar, and salt. However, the more specific recommendations to eat less meat, butter, and eggs and substitute nonfat milk for whole milk were most controversial. Many of the traditional messages of the past were now out of favor as were many cookbook authors and authorities that had been giving us nutritional advice for years. The warnings concerning eggs and milk even caused natural food buffs and vegetarians to reevaluate their diets. But, make no mistake about it, the dairy, meat, and egg producers were the most up in arms over this new advice.[27] The controversy did cause the committee to publish a revised version of the report later in 1977 but generally the thrust of the anti-fat and cholesterol message was not compromised in the second installment. The Dietary Goals were never declared an "official" government statement but it certainly jumpstarted the anti-fat movement, three years later in 1980 the United States Department of Agriculture joined the anti-fat crusade by publishing "Nutrition and Your Health: Dietary Guidelines for Americans." In 1984 the National Institute of Health chimed in with the recommendation that all Americans over age two should eat less fat.[28] At this point, although at least a portion of the scientific community was shaking their heads in disagreement, the fat was officially in the fire. Of course the food industry was licking their chops over the anticipation of the high profits from low-fat food marketing. As a consequence, many nutritional scientists have devoted their careers over the past few decades to showing scientifically what was already widely but prematurely accepted as fact by the U. S. government, media, low-fat food industry, and general public (i.e., dietary fat is scourge to modern humans). Although there have been many scientific attempts to find dangers in fat consumption, an abundance of scientific research still does not damn dietary fat as disease causing, and as described previously many types of dietary fat now have an extremely positive reputation in much of the scientific community. Harvard's Walter Willett recently conveyed in the January 2003 issue of *Scientific American* that this overall and total condemnation of dietary fat has occurred in part because authorities from the United States Department of Agriculture and "many nutritionists decided it would be too difficult to educate the public about these subtleties."[7]

Fat Restriction

There appear to be three somewhat separate views in the scientific literature regarding dietary fat but all claim to have science on their side. One segment clearly views all types of fat as a health menace, thus, they advocate fat restriction, the importance of low-fat diets for everyone, and replacing calories from dietary fat with carbohydrates. Critics would argue that these folks are guided by dogma more than science, however, this view may make intuitive sense. One reason why the low-fat hysteria has become so prominent and will likely be difficult to temper (should this be desirable) is because it makes intuitive sense that eating fat causes obesity and fatty buildup in arteries (i.e., we are what we eat). Most authorities who are familiar with fat consumption trends in the United States believe that dietary fat intake among Americans has decreased (at least as a percentage of total calories) over the last thirty years. The fat restrictors would be the first to say that this trend accounts for the reductions in the prevalence of heart disease in the United States now compared to several decades ago. On the other hand, it has been argued by some that heart disease death rates have declined in recent years primarily because doctors are treating the condition more successfully these days. Those who advocate fat restriction seem to be skeptical about the likelihood that some types of dietary fat are healthful concerning heart disease and cancer. Fat restrictors often cite research where extremely low-fat diets and exercise were reported to be associated with improved heart-health to support their views.[29] Further, the fat restrictors generally believe that dietary fat is primarily responsible for obesity, however, this is very controversial given that many experts suggest that dietary fat intake has gone down while at the same time (everyone agrees) that the average American has gotten fatter. This information provokes some fat restrictors to question whether or not fat consumption has actually decreased in the United States. Many researchers agree that our methods for measuring dietary fat consumption in our population are inexact.

Those who endorse fat restriction, which includes much of the general public, are likely to praise the use of fat substitutes, which have become very popular over the past couple of decades in the United States. Fat substitutes are frequently used in salad dressings, snacks, and dessert items (e.g., donuts) but some have reported that they are not necessarily low-calorie alternatives to standard products. In these reduced-fat or low-fat products, fat is often replaced with protein-based or carbohydrate-based ingredients. Most recently, Olestra was developed and marketed; Olestra is a synthetic compound that is resistant to digestive enzymes.[15] Incidentally, Olestra was discovered "serendipitously" in the 1960s while researchers were attempting to develop an easily digestible fat for premature infants but by accident created a form of fat that cannot be digested.[28] Given that the average American is fatter to-day compared to twenty years ago, more and more people are now questioning the effectiveness of these products as weight-reduc-tion aids.

Do some foods that are advertised as low fat really contain simi-lar amounts or even more calories than their higher-fat alterna-tives? A half dozen or so snack foods that were advertised as low fat were compared with their higher fat alternatives. In one case, the low-fat alternative was found to contain more calories per gram than the regular fat variety. However, unexpectedly the compari-sons revealed that the lower fat varieties of snack foods usually contained higher levels of other nutrients with negative reputations, i.e., salt and sugar, than the standard varieties. Further, some au-thorities claim that many of us tend to eat more of a food if we believe it to be low in fat, and that low-fat foods may contribute to type 2 diabetes (what used to be called adult-onset diabetes), the prevalence of which has increased in recent years. Thus, there are additional reasons to question whether or not low-fat foods are in fact healthful alternatives as many of us believe.

Is pork prohibition in our future? According to some authors who advocate fat restriction our government should intervene more strongly to change what we eat. One endorser of fat restriction who recently published a book entitled *The Politics of Dietary Fat* re-lated that government messages concerning the dangers of dietary fat have routinely lagged behind the incriminating scientific evi-dence against this nutrient. However, the sentiment that the gov-ernment has been irresponsibly sluggish about dietary fat warnings is not supported by many fat researchers, in fact, just the opposite, as previously stated several have suggested that the government leaped blindly on the anti-fat bandwagon. This particular anti-fat scholar perceives that the federal government is inconsistent re-garding its position on dietary fat. On the one hand the federal government promotes and subsidizes agricultural businesses (e.g., the dairy industry) which make high-fat products available in abun-dance and inexpensive for the American people: on the other hand the federal government publishes and disseminates information that advises Americans to reduce their dietary fat consumption. She went on to convey that it is clearly a necessity for the federal government to take further action to limit the availability and consumption of fat since, in her view, it is a leading contributor to disease and death in our society. According to some fat restrictors, one appropriate and long overdue way to rectify this perceived illogical and contradictory approach to dietary fat is for the federal government to change its emphasis regarding agricultural business so that it is less profitable for farmers to produce products that are deemed by some to be harmful to the public. Additionally, she suggested that other methods to reduce fat consumption may be justified, for example, taxing high-fat foods as we currently do tobacco products (often referred to as sin taxes). Further, modifying our food supply so that it contains less fat but remains tasty (e.g., adding air or water to food or using fat substitutes like olestra) is another common theme discussed in this text. Other more draconian measures could involve limiting or prohibiting the production, distribution, promotion, or sale of high-fat foods.[28] Similarly, it is noteworthy that apparently some ardent fat restrictors are eagerly awaiting a day when raising children with meat in the home will be considered child abuse.[30]

Although many of those who endorse fat restriction frequently warn Americans of the dangers of dietary fat as a promoter of diseases of the heart or vascular system, they also often express similar sentiments about the role of dietary fat in cancer development. An association between dietary fat and cancer in animals was first reported approximately one half century ago. However, much of this evidence associating dietary fat and cancer is highly controversial.[31] For example, nutritional researchers have known for quite some time that dramatic caloric restriction reduces cancer risk and increases longevity in lab animals. Thus, caloric restriction has been established, particularly in rodents, as a "powerful anti-carcinogen" because it reduces the risk of almost all types of cancer.[32] However, attempts to implicate specific dietary components (e.g., dietary fat or a subtype of fat) in cancer development, especially for humans, has met with less success. Some of the problems stem from the inability of investigators to accurately assess total caloric intake and fat consumption in epidemiological research. Also, finding correlations between cancer development and fat intake is not difficult, however, attributing a causal role to dietary fat would be considered by many to be an inappropriate, dangerous, and controversial leap.[31] For instance, total energy intake, exercise habits, body weight, fiber consumption, lack of some vitamin or mineral, or some unknown factor (either environmental or genetic) may explain such correlations and be the true villain. For example, it has been established that the act of cooking certain foods produces carcinogenic compounds and these compounds have been shown to be produce cancer in mice and rats.[33, 34] These cancer-promoting compounds may explain why "laboratory experimentation suggests that saturated fats are relatively poor cancer promoters"[35] while epidemiological research has implicated saturated fat in cancer development. However, one must always keep in mind that epidemiological research is all too often laden with problems and some would argue cannot be trusted.[36]

Somewhat surprising is the fact that animal studies have implicated certain polyunsaturated fatty acids as cancer promoters. For example, one of the essential fatty acids for humans (i.e., linoleic acid) has been found to increase the number and size of tumors in rodents.[11, 35] On the other hand, other polyunsaturated fats (e.g., the omega-3 fatty acids) have been found to decrease the size and number of tumors in animals. Epidemiological studies support the animal data in this case and suggest that omega-3 fatty acids protect against the development of cancers.[11, 35]

Thus, although fat restriction books directed at the lay audience often warn that, "There is no question that a high-fat diet increases the risk of many cancers, "[37] many in the scientific community are more cautious. Similarly, cancer research organizations (e.g., the American Institute for Cancer Research) have found no compelling nor even probable reason to believe that dietary fat causes cancer.[23] For instance, although some scientists believe that certain types of dietary fat may inhibit the growth of breast cancer, the best scientific information available indicates "overall, no relationship between fat and fat subtypes" for development of breast cancer in women or breast cancer mortality. The same can also be said for prostate cancer in men.[38]

Every previous researcher (besides Oakes and Slotterback) who has investigated gender differences in views of food healthfulness or who compared the types of foods that men and women eat have used this restriction perspective as the gold standard for healthy eating. In other words, researchers who compare men and women concerning healthy eating have traditionally accepted the fat-re-striction approach as some sort of hammered-in-stone manual describing how to be slim, healthy, and long lived. Without a doubt women, more than men, have assimilated the idea that fat restriction is healthful and that other nutrients are much less important. Thus, when researchers define healthy eating in terms of fat restriction women are always found to be very knowledgeable about healthy eating and conscientious regarding their diets compared to men. This fat-restriction perspective for health is accepted as sacred and factual, however, it is probably better described as theory with an intuitively sensible sounding ring and some supporting scientific evidence. Although the fat restriction message is zealously defended by many experts, the food industry, and lay people alike, below you will get a more detailed glimpse of the controversy surrounding dietary fat. Some would convey that fat-restriction theory is not standing up well with time. Perhaps, the potential merits of the anti-fat campaign were obscured and overstated to a degree that the message became harmful propaganda. Believe it or not, the American Heart Association (AHA) is now providing information about the possible dangers of low-fat diets. Such diets, according to the AHA, may increase coronary disease risk (e.g., by decreasing HDL cholesterol) in some people as well as promote obesity and malnutrition.[39]

Fat Replacement

A second, and perhaps growing, segment of the scientific community endorses fat replacement: this involves replacing dietary fat that has a negative reputation (i.e., saturated fat) with fat that has a more positive reputation (i.e., unsaturated fat), rather than replacing fat with carbohydrates. Those who endorse fat replacement argue that replacing saturated fat in our diets with carbohydrates contributes to an undesirable cholesterol profile (i.e., lowering levels of HDL, the molecule thought responsible for ridding the body of cholesterol). As described earlier in this chapter, those who espouse fat replacement are a dominant voice in the scientific literature as it pertains to the relationships between diet and disease. Further, many are a bit more skeptical regarding whether or not dietary fat consumption is primarily responsible for obesity in the United States. For example, those who endorse fat replacement are

more apt to attribute our health problems and obesity to our escalating consumption of refined carbohydrates (e.g., soda pop and
products made with white flour) and some claim that low-fat diets
actually promote obesity at least for many of us. One advocate of
fat replacement is Harvard's Walter Willett who recently conveyed
in *Scientific American* magazine that "no study has demonstrated
long-term benefits that can be directly attributed to a low-fat diet."[7]
Additionally, nutritional researchers from Harvard, who endorse
fat replacement, were recently quoted by CNN as saying the following, "You know what? Just like fats, there are good carbs and
there are bad carbs" and "You want to eat minimal amounts of
pasta, for example, or potatoes, things that are just starches and
don't have much else going for them."[40] Thus, some prestigious
advocates of fat replacement are now badmouthing the longtime-
lauded pasta and contributing to the negativity of the already ma-
ligned potato.

Fat Renegades

A third segment of the scientific community that is vocal about
dietary fat are those who are extremely skeptical about the reports
of dietary fat (of any type) as a silent assassin and contributor to
obesity. The government recommendations and warnings, which
were geared toward the entire American population, were, according to the fat renegades, inappropriate, extremely overstated, and
harmful given the fact that dietary fat is so important and that vast
amounts of scientific data do not support the hypothesis that even
saturated fat is worthy of its heinous reputation.[41] One writer who
has recently published at least two provocative accounts of the
problems with the low-fat message is Gary Taubes. One was published in the widely respected *Science* magazine in early 2001[23]
the other in the *New York Times Magazine* in mid 2002.[42] Taubes
and other fat renegades have indicated that the evidence which
supports the image of dietary fat (even saturated fat) as having a
capacity to snuff out human life is inconsistent, extremely weak,
and largely correlational, meaning that cause and effect cannot be
addressed and that other factors such as low fruit and vegetable
consumption are more likely responsible. Further, it has been suggested that of the evidence there is, much was obtained from examining men, thus, recommending dietary changes for women and

children is inappropriate and potentially harmful. For example, women who eat less meat may be at an increased risk for health problems like osteoporosis and anemia.[43] Another common theme is that low-fat diets may make heart disease less likely in middle-aged men but raise our susceptibility to other ailments (even other heart-related conditions).[44] The fact that some recent and widely respected research has found decreased likelihood of death from heart attacks while eating a Mediterranean diet but with no changes in cholesterol profiles has added fuel to the renegades' fire. Thus, the renegades are questioning the importance of the blood cholesterol profile as a measure of risk for dying from heart disease and they point out that attempts to lower blood cholesterol have, in some studies, been associated with increased overall death rates.[45] Further, the renegades are quick to point out that even the supposed harmful types of saturated fat (e.g., palmitic acid) have mixed (both good and bad) effects on blood cholesterol profiles anyway (i.e., raising both HDL and LDL).

Like most authorities, fat renegades accept that dietary fat consumption (as a percentage of total calories) has been significantly reduced in the United States in the last few decades but the renegades attribute reductions in heart disease to better treatment and less smoking, not less fatty diets. Why are Americans increasingly plump and diabetic? Well the renegades are not shy about placing the blame squarely on low-fat/high carbohydrate mania more than any other potential contributor (e.g., TV, fast food, increased portion sizes, or lack of exercise). They, with little reservation, endorse the hypothesis that high carbohydrate foods (with refined carbohydrates being worst), due to the fact that they are digested so easily and quickly, cause overeating and, ultimately over the long haul, diabetes.[42] Certainly, according to the United States Department of Agriculture, we are gobbling up more calories than ever before with the additional calories coming primarily in the form of carbohydrates.[18] The fat renegades are attacking the reputations of many foods that we have been led to believe are healthful over the past twenty-five years, for example, bagels, rice, pasta, juices, bread. As expected they view the recent explosion in soft drink, sports drink, and sugary tea and coffee consumption as an extremely negative trend, and as you likely would now predict, the lowly potato is at the top of their "don't do list."

Although the fat renegade perspective has much in common with the fat replacement viewpoint, those who favor the alternative and majority views on dietary fat (which have already been discussed) have been feuding with the renegades in *Science* magazine for the past few months. The opposition does not refute much of Taube's insights but has claimed that Taube's work promotes confusion which "does a disservice to the public health"[46] and according to other authorities "the article is misleading and counterproductive for public health policy to reduce dietary fat content."[47] Many Americans are confused about nutrition, but there is little reason to believe that the fat renegades deserve disproportionate blame.

Summary and Concluding Remarks

In this chapter, facts were provided that indicate the important roles of fat in the human body as well as in our diets. It is becoming accepted more and more (at least within the scientific community) that the initial condemnation of dietary fat as a killer was not based in good science and that the most persuasive messages against this nutrient, at least initially, came from our politicians and the food industry. Some of the most respected and often-quoted dietary-fat researchers in the world now acknowledge that the indiscriminate vilification of dietary fat over the years by the U.S. government, food industry, and other health experts was wrong and probably has done more harm than good. Although the lay community generally considers dietary fat of all types to be a pestilence, the scientific community is anything but united concerning their views about the benefits and dangers of the components of this nutrient and likely will continue to be at odds for quite some time. However, there seems to be a growing trend among scientists toward viewing consumption of some types of dietary fat as extremely important for health. A definitive study that would likely resolve some of these controversies is prohibitive because it would be extremely difficult, expensive, time consuming, and maybe even unethical. For example, to resolve whether saturated fat consumption really causes premature death, we could randomly divide a very large number of willing healthy people into groups (the most simple example would be a high-saturated-fat-diet group and a low-saturated-fat-diet group), give them routine physicals, and monitor their health until death. However, the problems would be staggering: it would take thousands of people, the study would last for many decades and would be enormously expensive, their diets would have to be similar in every other way except for saturated fat, it would be almost impossible to monitor the participants' diets to insure compliance, compliance would likely decrease for both groups over the years, and given that it is suspected that saturated fat is harmful it likely would be unethical to carry out such a study.

Thus, this is where our society appears to be regarding dietary fat. The nutritional scientists are divided and the majority of lay people are either accepting the fat restriction message as scripture (particularly women) or are confused and put off by the lack of consensus and contradictions regarding the dietary fat message. Aside from the charges made by the fat replacers and renegades, one could easily argue that the fat-restriction message, as it has been assimilated into the consciousness of most Americans, is irrational and an extremely narrow way to define healthy eating. Certainly there is likely no other nutrition message in American history that has impacted food reputations to the degree of the anti-fat crusade of the past several decades. Finally, there is likely no other nutritional issue that evokes the extreme emotional responses in Americans as does the fat controversy. Frequently, other political passions that are not directly related to nutrition (e.g., animal rights) contribute an added emotional charge to this issue.[48]

Notes

1. M. E. Oakes and C. S. Slotterback, What's in a name? A comparison of men's and women's judgements about food names and their nutrient contents, *Appetite* 36 (2001[b]), 29-40.
2. M. E. Oakes and C. S. Slotterback, Judgements of food healthfulness: food name stereotypes in adults over age 25, *Appetite* 37 (2001[c]), 1-8.
3. M. Eastwood, *Principles of human nutrition* (New York: Chapman and Hall 1997).
4. J. L Groff, S. S. Gropper, and S. M. Hunt, *Advanced nutrition and human metabolism* (New York: West Publishing Company 1995).
5. W. C. Willett, *Nutritional Epidemiology* (New York: Oxford University Press 1990).
   6. Willett, *Nutritional Epidemiology*, p. 333.
7. W. C. Willett and M. J. Stampfer, Rebuilding the food pyramid, *Scientific American* (January 2003), 64-71.
8. J. E. Vanderveen, The regulatory history for stearic acid, *The American Journal of Clinical Nutrition* 60 (1994), 983S-985S.
9. S. Renaud and D. Lanzmann-Petithory, Coronary heart disease: Dietary links and pathogenesis, *Public Health Nutrition* 4 (2001), 459-474.

10. C. von Schacky and J. Dyerberg, Omega-3 fatty acids: From Eskimos to clinical cardiology-what took us so long? *World Review of Nutrition Diet* 88 (2001), 90-99.
11. A. P. Simopoulos, The Mediterranean diet: What is so special about the diet of Greece? The scientific evidence, *Journal of Nutrition*, 131 (2001), 3065S-3073S.
12. D. Kromhout, Diet and cardiovascular disease, *The Journal of Nutrition, Health and Aging* 5 (2001), 144-149.
13. F. B. Hu, J. E. Manson, and W. C. Willett, Types of dietary fat and risk of coronary heart disease: A critical review, *Journal of the American College of Nutrition* 20 (2001), 5-19.
14. J. W. Santrock, *Children* 7ᵗʰ edition (New York: McGraw Hill 2003), 165.
15. E. N. McIntosh, *American food habits in historical perspective* (Westport, CT: Praeger 1995).
16. H. Levenstein, *Revolution at the table* (New York: Oxford University Press 1988), 21-22.
17. C. C. Furnas and S. M. Furnas, *Man, Bread and destiny*, (New York: Reynal and Hitchcock 1937).
18. USDA, Agriculture Fact Book 2000.
19. J. A. T. Pennington, *Bowes and Church's Food values of portions commonly used* (Philadelphia, PA: Lippincott 1998).
20. A. M. Katz, Trans-fatty acids and sudden cardiac death, *Circulation* 105 (2002), 669-671.
21. W. E. Conner and S. L. Conner, Should a low fat, high carbohydrate diet be recommended for everyone, *The New England Journal of Medicine* 337 (1997), 562-563.
22. T. Gordon, The diet-heart idea: Outline of a history, *American Journal of Epidemiology* 127 (1988), 220-225.
23. G. Taubes, The soft science of dietary fat, *Science* 291 (March, 2001), 2536-2545.
24. S. Brink, Unlocking the heart's secrets, *U.S. News and World Report* (September 1998), 58-66.
25. A. Keys, et al., *Seven countries: A multivariate analyses of death and coronary heart disease* (Cambridge, MA: Harvard University Press 1980).
26. A. Keys, et al, The diet and 15-year death rate in the seven countries study, *American Journal of Epidemiology* 124 (1986), 903-915.
27. H. Levenstein, *Paradox of plenty: A social history of eating in modern America* (New York: Oxford University Press 1993), 207-208.
28. L. S. Sims, *The politics of fat* (Armonk, NY: M. E. Sharpe 1998).
29. E. J. Schaefer, Lipoproteins, nutrition, and heart disease, *American Journal of Nutrition* 75 (2002), 191-212.
30. M. Stacey, *Consumed: Why Americans love, hate, and fear food* (New York: Simon and Schuster 1994), 171.
31. A.H. Lichtenstein, E. Kennedy, P. Barrier, D. Danford, et al., Dietary fat consumption and health/discussion, *Nutritional Reviews* 56 (1998) S3-S28.
32. The Council on Scientific Affairs, AMA, Diet and cancer: Where do matters stand? *Archives of Internal Medicine* 153 (1993) 50-56.
33. T. Shirai, et al., The prostate: A target for carcinogenicity of 2-amino-1-methyl-6-phenylimidazo [4, 5-b]pyridine (PhIP) derived from cooked foods, *Cancer research*, 57 (1997) 195-198.
34. T. Sugimura, Carcinogenicity of mutagenic heterocyclic amines formed during the cooking process, *Mutation Research* 150 (1985) 33-41.
35. J. H. Weisburger, Dietary fat and risk of chronic disease: Mechanistic insight from experimental studies, *Journal of the American Dietetic Association* 97 supplement (1997) S16-S23.

36. J. H. Weisburger, Dietary fat and risk of chronic disease: Mechanistic insight from experimental studies, *Journal of the American Dietetic Association* 97 supplement (1997) S16-S23.

37. J. Fuhrman, *Eat to live: The revolutionary formula for fast and sustained weight loss* (New York: Little, Brown, and Company 2003), 134.

38. M. A. Moyad, Dietary fat reduction to reduce prostate cancer risk: Controlled enthusiasm, learning a lesson from breast or other cancers, and the big picture, *Urology* 59 (Supplement 4A, April, 2002), 51-62.

39. R. M. Krauss, et al. AHA dietary guidelines revision 2000: A statement for healthcare professionals from the nutrition committee of the American Hear Association, *Circulation* 102 (2000) 2284-2299.

40. CNN.com—Elizabeth Cohen: The Skinny on 'good fats'—July 8, 2002: Http// www.cnn.com/2002/HE...fitness/07/08/cohen.fat.otsc/index.ht

41. U. Ravnskov, The questionable role or saturated and polyunsaturated fatty acids in cardiovascular disease, *Clinical Epidemiology* 51 (1998), 443-460.

42. G. Taubes, What if fat doesn't make you fat? *New York Times Magazine* (July 7, 2002).

43. P. A. Crotty, *Good Nutrition?*, St. Leonards, Australia (1995), 62.

44. B. A. Golomb, Dietary fats and heart disease—dogma challenged, *Clinical Epidemiology* 51 (1998), 461-464.

45. D. A. Atrens, The questionable wisdom of low-fat diet and cholesterol reduction, *Social Science and Medicine* 39 (1994), 433-447.

46. S. M. Grundy, Dietary fat: at the heart of the matter, *Science* 293 (August 2001), 801-802.

47. A.Astrup, J. O. Hill, and W. H. M. Saris, Dietary fat: at the heart of the matter, *Science*, 293 (August 2001), 803.

48. M. Stacey, *Consumed*: 157.

4

The Worth of One's Salt

The Reputation of Salt

As described previously, when judging the health value of a food (e.g., a food name like "apple") only the fat content, and no other nutrient characteristic, of the food predicted its healthfulness rating for young and older women. However, for men of all ages both fat content and amounts of vitamins and minerals were predictive of ratings of food healthfulness. There was no sign that the sodium content of food was used when judging the healthfulness of food names. Thus, it appears that the sodium content of a food has little impact on a food's reputation (i.e., as observed when evaluating the healthfulness of food names).[1, 2] On the other hand, when rating the healthfulness of a food's description (i.e., the amounts of calories, fat, protein, fiber, cholesterol, and sodium as well as vitamins and minerals in a food) without knowledge of the food's name sodium content was somewhat predictive of health ratings for older respondents but not for younger men and women. As the amount of sodium indicated in a food description increased the health rating of the food description decreased for the older respondents. Thus, there is little doubt that sodium itself does have a negative reputation at least among older people in the United States.[2] However, fat has a more negative reputation: fat content was most highly correlated with the health ratings of food descriptions for men and women of all ages. Finally, when asked to select the food characteristic most important for health from a list that was provided, more elderly people than any other age group selected sodium content. However, freshness, fat content, and naturalness (in that order) were more often considered most important for health by elderly respondents.[3]

When rating the healthfulness of food names and descriptions, it seemed surprising initially that older adults rated the descriptions of certain foods, for example, tuna, Cheerios, bagel, hotdog, fried chicken, hamburger, and cottage cheese as less healthful than did college-aged adults (the name ratings for these foods did not vary between the two age groups). Then we realized that all of these foods have high levels of sodium and that the older respondents were attending to the sodium content provided in the food descriptions more than were the younger participants. Some high sodium foods (e.g., bagels and Cheerios) have a very good reputation (i.e., high healthfulness rating for their name) in our society primarily because they are low in fat but the amount of sodium indicated in the food descriptions caused these foods' descriptions to be rated lower in terms of healthfulness by older people. Thus, although sodium has a negative reputation among older women, the reliance on food reputations when selecting foods to eat likely causes them to choose low-fat foods with little or no consideration of other food characteristics like sodium content.[2]

Salty Facts?

Although sometimes the terms salt and sodium are used interchangeably, salt is actually composed of both sodium and chloride. More specifically, by weight, salt is 40 percent sodium and 60 percent chloride. The average American eats about 9 grams of salt daily, an estimated 80 percent of which is non-discretionary meaning that it comes from processed foods. The recommended intake of salt according to the United States government is now six grams daily, which is estimated to be at least ten times more than we actually need. There appears to be some uncertainty about the amount of salt that is necessary for humans given that researchers have reported that one primitive tribe in South America sustained themselves on as little as one-twentieth of a gram of salt daily.[4] Several sources indicated that we need about half of a gram of salt daily but at least one other source suggested that one-fourth of a gram may be sufficient.[5]

Americans are not the biggest salt gluttons in the world: people living in certain areas of Japan and Portugal reportedly eat between twenty and thirty grams of salt daily.[4] Only about 20 percent of the salt that Americans eat is discretionary (i.e., what we actually add during cooking or at the table), the rest (80 percent) as mentioned previously, comes from processed foods like cereals, processed meat (e.g., ham, pepperoni, salami, and hotdogs), cheeses, and canned products (e.g., soups). Restaurant food is often loaded with sodium, for example, a fried seafood platter has almost double the recommended daily value for sodium and this is just one meal.[6] Salt and other sodium containing compounds are used in the food industry to enhance flavor of foods, to improve the texture and mouth feel of foods, and for inhibiting spoilage (e.g., sodium suppresses growth of dangerous microorganisms like those that cause botulism).[7] The food industry has received pressure over the past few of decades to reduce sodium content in their products and apparently they quietly have done so: from 1983 to 1994 sodium content dropped 10-15 percent in processed foods.[8]

Why is Sodium Necessary in Our Diets?

Sodium constitutes about .2 percent of the body, most of it is found in fluids outside of cells. Sodium is important for regulating the levels of body fluids and in maintaining acid-base balance in the body. Further, sodium plays a role in regulating the activity of the heart and in metabolism of protein and carbohydrates.[7] Nervous system communication is to a large extent electrical and sodium is an essential mineral contributing to each of the billions of electrical signals that occur each minute to keep us alive and functioning. In fact, local anesthetics like novocaine, when injected into isolated parts of our body, work by inhibiting sodium's capacity to enter nervous system cells in the area around the injection site. Thus, these drugs reduce the electrical activity in the part of the body affected and inhibit our abilities to detect sensory signals (e.g., pain and taste) as well as our capacity to control the muscles of the effected region. The influence on muscle control explains why we may slobber and have a difficult time talking after receiving local anesthetics at the dentist. Below, a description of the devastating consequences that result when sodium becomes depleted throughout our bodies will be provided.

Salt makes up about 0.9 percent of the blood. When salt becomes too diluted (i.e., less concentrated) in our bodies due to disease or too little salt in the diet accompanied by extreme sweating, diarrhea, or drinking lots of water, our lives are in jeopardy. This condition is known as hyponatremia. When this condition results from drinking too much water it is sometimes referred to as water intoxication. We are more susceptible to this condition when we are babies: for this reason, pediatricians now advise caregivers to avoid giving plain water in bottles to babies when they are not yet eating solid foods.[9] Additionally, although healthy babies are born with a swimming reflex that may allow them to keep their heads above water briefly when placed in a swimming pool they may swallow excessive amounts of water which could result in water intoxication.[10] Water intoxication can occur at any age if a dehydrated person is not given appropriate treatment. In fact, use of the drug ecstasy has been associated with extreme dehydration. Apparently when ecstasy users respond to their thirst by drinking fluids with little or no sodium deaths have occurred due to water intoxication. However, water intoxication occurs most frequently among schizophrenics, possibly as a result of the disease itself or some interaction with the medications. Schizophrenic patients have been known to drink as much ten gallons of water a day and if denied water they will resort to drinking from aquariums, toilets, and radiators.[11] Thus, we think of water as the most benign substance that we can take into our bodies, however, when consumed in high amounts without accompanying sodium, negative health consequences can result.

Blood Pressure

As most of us know sodium consumption has been implicated in high blood pressure, but what is blood pressure? First, I have come to realize that many of my students seem to think that blood saturates all of the tissues in our bodies, that is, they do not realize that blood should only be found in blood vessels. Many students are surprised to find out that adult humans only have about a gallon to a gallon and half of blood in their bodies and if blood is leaking (or more aptly squirting) out of blood vessels this indicates a problem (i.e., hemorrhage). Blood pressure refers to the force that blood exerts on our blood vessels as it circulates in our bodies. It has been known for at least several hundred years that blood circulates under pressure: in 1733 one curious fellow stuck a tube in the carotid artery of a horse and observed how the blood rushed into the tube and pulsated up and down with each heart beat. However, although the device for measuring blood pressure (called a sphygmomanometer) was developed in 1834, it was not until the twentieth century that we developed the capacity to reliably measure blood pressure and ultimately determine that high blood pressure was correlated with negative health consequences.[5]

The first sound that medical staff hear when measuring our blood pressure indicates the systolic pressure. Systolic pressure reflects the degree of resistance (i.e., elasticity) in blood vessels during heartbeats. The diastolic pressure (second number) reflects the rigidity of blood vessels between heartbeats when the heart is relaxing. It may seem somewhat paradoxical but when it comes to blood pressure "normal" does not necessarily mean "good" or "optimal" for the heart and vascular system. Most middle-aged men have a systolic blood pressure between 120-129 (normal), a level that is correlated with increased incidence of heart attack and stroke compared to a systolic pressure below 110. In fact, somewhat different than what was conveyed in the last chapter about cholesterol, no one disputes that as blood pressure increases death and disease risk also escalate. However the vast majority of people who experience a heart attack or stroke do not have high blood pressure, defined as 140 and above for systolic pressure and 90 and above for diastolic pressure.[12]

By far the most common type of hypertension (about 95 percent of cases) is termed essential or primary hypertension and refers to high blood pressure with no known cause. Essential hypertension is characterized by a gradual increase in blood pressure as we age. The contribution of dietary salt to essential hypertension is a controversial topic but certainly most experts would agree that increased salt intake exacerbates the problem in some of us. The more rare form of hypertension, called secondary hypertension, is due to some identifiable disease process often involving the kidneys or adrenal glands: dietary salt often raises blood pressure in people who have these sorts of diseases. Essential hypertension is thought to contribute to disease in several different organ systems including diseases of the heart, kidney, and cerebrovascular system (the latter in this case meaning a stroke).[13] Further, cross-sectional studies of blood pressure where, for example, the blood pressure of 20 year olds were compared to seventy year olds led many to assume that an individual's blood pressure tended to increase with age. However, longitudinal studies, which involved keeping track of a person's blood pressure over several decades, have revealed that only in a portion of the population do we see blood pressure escalating as they get older.[14]

How did Salt Fall into Disrepute?

Salt was first implicated in high blood pressure back in 1904 when researchers working in France demonstrated that high salt diets raised blood pressure in most of the six hypertensive patients that were examined. Although this study was the first to implicate salt intake, other investigators who attempted to replicate these findings often found that manipulations involving dietary salt had little effect on blood pressure in the patients that they studied. Thus, the notion that salt caused hypertension never really came in favor until several decades later: the prevailing theory was that excessive protein intake caused high blood pressure.[15] In the early twentieth century, there was considerable controversy concerning what the optimal levels of protein should be in the diet. One eccentric, at least by today's standards, who advocated low protein diets for a variety of health reasons was Horace Fletcher. Fletcher was an early twentieth-century health and diet guru whose notoriety at the time was likely eclipsed only by the illustrious and irrepressible Dr. Kellogg. Fletcher was known not only for low protein diets, he was also most obsessed with thorough mastication (chewing food until it was of fluid consistency). Low protein consumption and for some what came to be known as "Fletcherizing" (i.e., extreme chewing of edibles) were effective treatments for all sorts of internal disorders including hypertension and, of course, dyspepsia. Fletcher's message was particularly compelling because as a middle-aged man he could reportedly out perform college athletes in feats of strength and endurance. Finally, although at risk of seeming indelicate to the reader, many experts at the time were apparently struck by the lack of odors emanating from Fletcher's stools. Horace gladly accommodated these captivated and devoted professional followers as it concerned this fascination by occasionally mailing his stools to them.[16] How and where Horace died seems to be debated among historians. One historian indicated that Horace died in 1919 in Battle Creek from complications of malnutrition.[17] However, another source conveyed that Fletcher died in Europe and made no reference to malnutrition.[18]

Although the "protein intoxication" theory prevailed well into the 1930s, there were at least occasional studies involving salt manipulations on high blood pressure throughout the 1920s. One team of investigators publishing in 1929 reported increases in blood pressure in most of the fifty patients who had sought medical treatment for a variety of health problems (e.g., asthma, Parkinson's disease, heart disease, and even menopause) but instead of treatment were given three teaspoons of salt daily for one month. It is likely that the methodology of this particular study would be appropriately challenged if attempted today due to ethical concerns among other things. These patients, most of whom had serious health problems, were given no medications, the authors feared that drugs "might interfere with our experiment." Further, many of the patients had assorted problems associated with downing the required three teaspoons of salt daily, for example, some patients just conveyed their revulsion while others became nauseous.[19]

Most of those who were researching the effects of salt intake on blood pressure in the first decade or so of the twentieth century focused on the importance of the chloride portion that makes up salt rather than the sodium. It was not until the early 1920s that anyone even gave much consideration to the notion that the sodium component in salt may influence blood pressure. Throughout the 1920s and 30s a few authorities were advocating moderate salt restriction for hypertension but by the mid 1940s salt restriction had fallen out of favor once again and was nowhere to be seen in the medical literature.[20] For example, one notable researcher concluded in 1945 that any positive results on blood pressure that had been attributed to salt restriction were in fact due to bed rest or constant medical attention (i.e., what we now call the placebo effect). It was well known even in the early twentieth century that blood pressure readings were extremely susceptible to both suggestion and what was called "spontaneous variation, " resulting from a variety of more or less unknown influences.[20] Their wisdom is still sound today, when evaluating blood pressure, several readings are required due to the fact that a single measure is an unreliable predictor of the usual blood pressure in a person.

The research that revived the sodium hypertension hypothesis was initiated in the mid-1940s by Wallace Kempner who oddly enough emphasized protein reduction rather than limiting salt intake. Kempner placed 500 hypertensive patients on a rice and fruit diet that involved dramatic limitations in consumption of protein, fat, cholesterol, salt, and calories. Kempner even limited the fluid intake in the patients he examined. However, the diet was high in potassium.[21] Such an extreme diet, lacking in amino acids, fatty acids, and certain minerals would not have been conducive to good health and a long life and several participants did die during the study. However, Kempner reported reductions in blood pressure and improvements in health for many of the patients as well as (no surprise) weight loss.[22] Other investigators who subsequently used the Kempner approach, which became the standard hypertension treatment in the late 1940s and early 50s, ultimately focused on the extreme sodium restriction as the effective feature of the diet for reducing blood pressure. No reason was given concerning why sodium was implicated more than any other characteristic of the diet. Extreme sodium restriction was the rule for most of these studies, in fact, some investigators concluded that severe sodium restriction was often necessary to lower blood pressure in hypertensive patients and that moderate sodium restriction was useless.[22] It is amazing that the Kempner diet was viewed as a success even in terms of its ability to reduce blood pressure: objective evaluation of the diet has revealed that perhaps 50 percent of the hypertensive subjects did not respond to this harsh diet.[23] Further, although only hypertensive patients were examined in many of these early studies involving extreme salt restriction, some authors did report that those without elevated blood pressure were most likely to develop "incapacitating" and "dangerous" symptoms when denied salt (specifically what these symptoms were was not mentioned).[24] The advent of oral diuretic drugs to treat high blood pressure, which occurred in the mid-1950s, mercifully pushed the Kempner diet out of fashion. However, the increasing awareness of adverse side effects from blood pressure medications has revived dietary salt restriction in the past few decades.[25]

The major champion of salt reduction for many years was physician and researcher Lewis Dahl. In fact, Dahl was really the first person to formally proclaim that salt causes hypertension in humans. Dahl reported starting back in the 1950s (and continuing until his death in the mid 1970s) that average sodium intake in a population was predictive of the prevalence of high blood pressure in a population, that is, as average sodium consumption increased in a population blood pressure also increased. The value of such studies in contributing to our understanding of the role of salt on blood pressure, according to many experts nowadays, is negligible given the inaccurate assessments of salt intake (most were based on guesses) and the likelihood that other dietary factors or social (e.g., obesity) and genetic factors could account for the findings.[26] Dahl is also noted for his work with animals, this primarily involved the development of a rodent model for hypertension. Through selective breeding of rats Dahl developed a strain that became hypertensive when fed salt (i.e., salt sensitive rats). However, it was not easy to make these rats hypertensive, they had to be fed huge amounts of salt, the equivalent to fifty times more than the average American consumes daily. For reasons such as this, many salt authorities question whether this or any other animal research is particularly helpful and relevant for understanding human essential hypertension.[27]

What has been described thus far gives a glimpse of the scientific evidence against salt in the 1970s when recommendations concerning lowering salt intake began to be disseminated by national health agencies. As was previously described for dietary fat, there was no definitive or monumental scientific discovery that preceded the United States government's initial warnings and recommendations concerning reductions of salt intake. Instead, a shift in the political wind brought this issue to our consciousness. For example, the same senate committee, chaired by George McGovern, that threw fat into the fire opted to toss salt in also.

A subsequent famous and notable or, more appropriately in the views of some, infamous and notorious scientific study that contributed to the development of salt's reputation (at least among scientists) is known in the scientific literature as the Intersalt study. Intersalt was designed to compare salt consumption and blood pressure among fifty-two different populations around the world without the methodological flaws of previous studies. The Intersalt investigators reported a weak correlation between blood pressure and salt intake across all of the 10,000 or so participants that were examined. In the view of many salt authorities, the results suggested that dramatic cuts in salt intake would result in only small reductions in blood pressure (i.e., on average a 2.2 point drop in systolic pressure and 0.1 drop in diastolic pressure). Further, the Intersalt folks reported an association between salt intake in populations and escalation of blood pressure with age. The latter of these two findings sparked an extreme controversy in the literature, which will described a bit later.[27]

Two recent studies that have provided insight into the role of sodium on high blood pressure go by the name DASH (Dietary Approaches to Stop Hypertension). The results of both studies have received a great deal of positive press with much praise coming from our own federal government. Both studies examined those with normal blood pressure and those with high blood pressure. The first DASH study was published in 1997 and involved no manipulations of salt intake. In fact, the original DASH study was designed to insure that salt intake was uniform for all participants and that body weight did not change throughout the study. One group was fed a typical American diet for eight weeks (control diet), a second group was given a diet rich in fruits and vegetables and fewer sweets but was otherwise similar to the control diet for the same period of time (fruit and vegetable diet), and a third group was fed a low-fat diet rich in fruits, vegetables, and low-fat dairy products for eight weeks (DASH diet). Generally, the results were impressive: the DASH diet reduced blood pressure more than the control or fruit and vegetable diets. The fruit and vegetable diet was less impressive but generally did reduce blood pressure compared to the control diet. Those with hypertension got the most blood-pressure-lowing benefits from the DASH diet. Further, the results did not seem to rankle anyone. In fact, although the findings from the original DASH study implied nothing positive or negative about salt, many of those who were skeptical about recommendations to lower sodium consumption applauded the study because, at least to them, it took the emphasis off salt and on to other dietary factors (e.g., too little calcium in our diets). However, it is impossible to know what characteristics or combinations of characteristics were responsible for the blood pressure lowering effects of the DASH diet The DASH diet was low in fat (27 percent of total calories) and cholesterol compared to the control diet but higher in almost everything else (e.g., protein, fiber, and most vitamins and minerals).[28]

The second edition of DASH was published in January of 2001 and did involve manipulations of sodium intake. One group was fed a typical American diet (control diet) and another the DASH diet for ninety days. Both diet groups were fed low salt diets (about three grams of salt daily) for thirty days, moderate salt diets (about six grams of salt daily) for thirty days, and high salt diets (about nine grams of salt daily which is typical for most Americans) for thirty days. Blood pressure was measured during the final few days of each thirty-day period. As was found for the original DASH study, the DASH diet lowered blood pressure compared to those fed the control diet. However, additionally, for this second study the DASH investigators found that concentrations of salt in the diet (low, moderate, and high) also influenced blood pressure. Blood pressure dropped most for those eating the DASH diet when they were fed the lowest concentration of salt. Once again those with hypertension were helped most. The authors concluded with no reservations that most Americans should reduce their salt intake and pursue a more DASH-like diet in order to lower their blood pressure.[29] Our federal government is now supporting these recommendations. As you might expect, this study has ruffled some feathers. Critics have pointed out that for those with normal blood pressure and who are eating the DASH diet, the most severe salt restriction had almost no impact on blood pressure.[30] Also, skeptics have emphasized that there was an overrepresentation of subjects in the study who one would expect to respond to low-salt diets: proportionately speaking there were more African Americans, hypertensives, and overweight subjects in the DASH study than exist in the American population.[31] Finally, the study was short and strictly controlled: similar results may be hard to achieve in the real world. For example, the subjects either ate their meals at the clinic or took clinic food home with them.

The Salt Suppressors versus Salt Subverts

Generally, there appears to be two opinions regarding the wisdom of public health initiatives to reduce salt intake in the United States. Salt suppressors are those who view salt as a deadly white powder and endorse the notion that all Americans should reduce their sodium consumption. Reducing salt intake, according to the suppressors, will benefit many (perhaps everybody) and harm no one. Further, targeting the entire American population is more desirable and effective than attempting to identify those at risk, which really is not possible at this time, and directing dietary advice only to these people. Since most of the dietary sodium that we eat is non-discretionary meaning that it is already present in processed foods that we purchase and eat (as opposed to discretionary salt which is added during cooking or at the table), salt suppressors are asking or perhaps in some cases demanding that the food industry reduce concentrations of salt in processed foods.[32] Some investigators in the salt suppressor camp are encouraging the food industry to gradually rather than abruptly lower the salt concentration of foods. They admit that in the real world abrupt changes in dietary salt concentrations of the magnitude used in the most recent DASH study are almost intolerable for people. Further, people tend to compensate for abrupt dietary salt reductions by adding fat to their diet. Therefore, these folks predict that with gradual reductions in our food's salt concentration adaptation will be much easier: once adaptation occurs to low-salt diets, our current American fare will likely be perceived as intolerably salty.[33]

Salt suppressors are emphatic about educating people about the salt content of foods, how to decrease salt intake, and what they perceive to be the obvious and undeniable dangers of excessive salt consumption. The debate concerning the risks and benefits of eating less salt have been characterized as "false" and "synthetic" by those who advocate a universal "pulling in the reins" concerning salt consumption. In almost every book or article encountered that touched on the controversy surrounding limiting salt consumption in our population, those who endorsed the salt suppression perspective were quick and vehement in stating that there really is no controversy. In other words, salt suppressors seem to feel that all of those who are opposed to salt restriction on a national scale are cruel, irresponsible, and subversive puppets who have been bought by the salt, processed food, or even dairy industries. Salt suppressors routinely liken the salt industry and to some extent processed food manufacturers to the tobacco industry: the suppressors relate that the debate is a masquerade motivated by greed and created by the salt and processed food industries to purposely distort what they see as irrefutable evidence that our current level of salt consumption is ending our lives prematurely. This analogy between the food and tobacco industries appears again and again in the literature.[27, 34]

As alluded to above, those who are critical of the food industry's reliance on salt have stated that the motives behind the high salt content in processed foods are based in greed. For example, salt increases the weight of foods and the food industry is concerned that the public may not be enthusiastic about paying the same amount for low salt foods that weigh much less. Also, the fact that salty foods induce thirst is important: beverage manufacturers often own companies that make salty snacks. Thus, the beverage industry is dependent upon salty foods to maintain sales of soft drinks and alcoholic beverages.[34]

Some salt suppressors support salt substitution, this often involves substituting sodium for some other mineral, for example, potassium chloride is most commonly used. However, potassium for some people, particularly when used in excess can have harmful side effects. Several incidences of poisoning with the salt substitute potassium chloride have been documented involving people of all ages.[35] It is essential that any salt substitute be carefully evaluated for several years before being widely marketed. The first account that I could find involving the use of what we now know to be dangerous salt substitutes extends back to the first half of the twentieth century. During the 1940s lithium chloride was employed as a salt substitute for people with heart disease, in terms of flavor it reportedly worked well as a salt substitute. However, it had one serious drawback, it is fairly toxic and widespread use of lithium for this purpose resulted in illness and even death. Thus, the medical community was forced to abandon the use of lithium chloride as a salt substitute but lithium is still used to treat certain mental illnesses. In fact, as critics of salt reduction have suggested, reduced dietary sodium can cause retention of lithium in the body which can lead to toxic reactions in those taking the drug.[36]

What sorts of choices do shoppers have regarding low- or reduced-sodium snack foods? Surprisingly, especially when you consider the high numbers of elderly shoppers in the area, there were not many reduced-sodium foods available in the super market that we frequent. Of those low- or reduced-sodium snack foods found either potassium chloride was used as a salt substitute or nothing at all. Also, several of these modified-sodium foods had higher amounts of calories per serving than the identical regular sodium alternative. It has been reported that the food industry has made genuine efforts to introduce low-sodium products, however, many of these products have been withdrawn because the public will not purchase them.[37]

Salt suppressors accept that salt contributes to all of the diseases of the heart, kidney, and central nervous system that have been associated with high blood pressure. Additionally, the salt suppressors believe that salt contributes to certain diseases that may be independent of its effects on blood pressure, for example enlargement of the heart, stroke, stomach cancer, kidney stones, asthma, and osteoporosis.[38, 39] Also, another potential positive effect from limiting salt intake reductions in the amount of medication necessary to control blood pressure.

Salt subverts are those who believe that any attempt at reducing salt consumption throughout the general population in the United States is not justified and may in fact be detrimental to health. As one might expect the salt subverts are often offended by the suppressor's depiction of them as slimy disreputable thugs who are invariably on the food industry's payroll. Many subverts emphasize that for some (perhaps most) people salt intake (even at high doses) has very little impact on blood pressure. Further, subverts point out that salt restriction in people with normal blood pressure has been shown repeatedly to have very small (if any) effects on blood pressure even after extreme reductions in sodium intake. According to the salt subverts, at best salt restriction has a beneficial impact primarily for older people and those with hypertension. Also, the subverts often emphasize that reductions in blood pressure by limiting salt intake have been shown to be hard to sustain over a long period of time.[40] However, their opponents, the salt suppressors often respond by indicating that even small downward shifts in blood pressure in a population can cause more dramatic reductions in incidence of death from stoke and heart disease in a population.

Salt subverts often emphasize that other methods to decrease blood pressure are likely more effective and safer than limiting salt intake. Weight loss, exercise, and reduced alcohol consumption, for example, are often mentioned by both suppressors and subverts as being helpful for blood pressure reduction. Further, dietary changes that do not involve salt reduction are often supported by salt subverts: some emphasize increasing potassium consumption which has been shown to lower blood pressure in some studies. One group of investigators endorses eating more calcium rich foods to lower blood pressure. More rarely, other minerals like magnesium are touted for blood pressure reduction and even omega-3 fatty acids.[41-43]

Salt suppressors, when arguing their case and seemingly as a last resort, often state that salt reduction won't hurt anybody and will benefit many. On the other hand, some salt subverts claim that reducing salt consumption may cause health problems, some of which no one could predict beforehand. It has, in fact, been shown repeatedly that reductions in salt intake will increase blood pressure in some people, even among those who are already hypertensive. This heterogeneity in blood pressure response to dietary salt manipulations is somewhat problematic for those who endorse universal salt reduction.[23, 44] Further, other unanticipated health problems with lowering the sodium concentration of foods are possible. For example, a well-meaning attempt to lower the salt content of infant formula resulted in an unintended chloride deficiency in babies.[45] Additionally, results from one study suggested that low-sodium diets may contribute to chronic fatigue syndrome.[46]

Beyond this, is there any evidence available now suggesting that salt reduction is harmful? Yes, there is some evidence, however, what little evidence there is can be characterized as extremely weak. There are very few published studies which suggest that salt restriction is harmful: only about three or four published studies were found that expressed this message. The web site for the Salt Institute, an organization that represents the salt industry and is no doubt an archenemy of all salt suppressors, listed additional studies that suggested negative consequences from salt reduction but these studies have not been published and likely never will be. Salt subverts argue that the reason for the paltry number of published studies can be attributed to the fact that the subject has only rarely and recently been examined, which is probably true. Salt subverts are quick to point out that low blood pressure may be common in primitive societies where very little salt is consumed but it also should be noted that these people tend to die much younger compared to those of us in the United States. The methodology for the few studies that do report health problems with limiting salt intake have been widely criticized. Further, the interpretations of some of the findings have struck some salt authorities as being farfetched and blatantly slanted toward the salt-subvert perspective. For example, one group of investigators reported reductions in both coronary heart disease mortality and death from all causes in those who reported eating more salt. However, additionally in this study it was reported that people who consumed diets with high concentrations of salt were more likely to succumb to coronary heart disease. The investigators concluded that based on these findings recommendations to alter salt consumption in the general population are not justified. Interestingly, high absolute amounts of salt consumed predicted less death in this study. One reasonable interpretation coming from critics is that healthy active people eat more food and, thus, as a consequence they consume a bit more salt. Further, the fact that high concentrations of reported dietary salt intake predicted heart disease death may suggest, among other things, potential problems with salt: but, the investigators were not able to acknowledge this possibility in the published study.[47] On the other hand, the salt subverts appear to be accurate in that, as things stand now, there is not compelling evidence that eating lots of salt causes disease or premature death. As was indicated for dietary fat consumption, a definitive study on the effects of salt intake on disease and death has never been done. Curiously, one authority actually offered, then dismissed, the idea of introducing abundant amounts of salt to a primitive low-salt consuming society for a period of time then assessing their blood pressure.[48]

Areas of Controversy

As described above, the main controversy that appears again and again in the literature involves whether or not population-wide sodium restriction is justified and likely beneficial or instead unnecessary and potentially harmful. Several smaller controversies exist that make a definitive answer to the main controversy somewhat elusive. As one group who reviewed the salt and hypertension literature indicated a few years back, convincing scientific arguments can be made either in support of salt restriction in the general population or to refute this position.[49]

What is the mechanism that explains how sodium increases blood pressure in some people? Although giving either animals or humans large quantity of sodium tends to increase blood volume (i.e., causing more blood to circulate in our blood vessels) and causes a transitory change in blood pressure, a mechanism to explain how salt might contribute to essential hypertension has been elusive given that most folks with essential hypertension do not have an increased blood volume. Thus, some experts hypothesize that chronic high salt consumption, through some unknown mechanism, may increase blood pressure by influencing the characteristics of blood vessel walls (e.g., causing constriction of the vessels) resulting in more resistance in blood flow through the blood vessels.[50] Individual variation in the kidneys' capacity to expel salt from the body, according to some authorities, may partially explain why some people are more susceptible to heightened blood pressure than others due to our salty diets.[51] In fact, although the entire concept is definitely controversial, the terms "salt resistant" and "salt sensitive" are often encountered in the literature. At least in theory, "salt resistant" people are those whose blood pressure is relatively insensitive to abrupt changes in salt intake while "salt sensitive" individuals are those who after abrupt changes in salt intake experience more dramatic increases in blood pressure. The controversies surrounding this issue involve the following: (1) there is no clear distinction between the two groups; (2) some people may appear salt sensitive on one occasion and salt resistant on another; (3) although some people believe that salt sensitive people are likely to develop hypertension later in life, there is really no evidence that these blood pressure fluctuations due to abrupt changes in sodium intake are helpful at all in predicting how someone will respond to a lifetime's exposure to sodium.[32, 52] Regardless of the controversy, the term "salt sensitive" is widely used: salt sensitivity is thought to be most common among black Americans and the elderly.[26]

In fact, a somewhat chilling theory has been proposed to explain why black Americans are more often found to be salt sensitive. It has been hypothesized that the hardships involving the transport of Africans to the western hemisphere for purposes of slavery might be responsible for the increased salt sensitivity and hypertension observed in black Americans. It has been estimated that 12 million black people were transported from western Africa to North and South America between 1500 and 1800. However, between capture and arrival in the western hemisphere their numbers were decimated with as many as 40-50 percent perishing during the journey. Some died on forced 100-200 mile marches to the West Coast of Africa after capture. Still more expired while residing in the crowded unventilated huts that served as cages awaiting the ocean voyage. However, the majority who perished succumbed during the ocean voyage. The dead and dieing were cavalierly thrown overboard while still in chains presumably, according to one source, to eagerly awaiting sharks. The causes of death varied, a few died from infection, some took their own life, but most died from illnesses related to dehydration from diarrhea and excessive heat. Thus, some hypothesize that those who were able to retain salt in their bodies had a potentially lifesaving advantage that allowed them to more likely endure these hardships and of course they would be the ancestors of many black Americans today. Essentially the ability to keep salt in the body would have been a blessing then but a curse nowadays due to the abundance of salty fare in our modern American diet. [53, 54]

As described previously, for some of us blood pressure increases as we get older: the authors of the Intersalt study implicated high salt consumption as the culprit. The extent to which sodium consumption over a lifetime interacts with genetics or some disease process to produce essential hypertension in a person has been an area of extreme debate. One of the many controversial aspects of the Intersalt study involved a strong tendency, according to the authors of the study, for blood pressure to increase with age in populations where sodium consumption is high. The Intersalt investigators were attempting to make the case that high salt consumption over many years likely causes blood pressure to increase with age. However, this interpretation of the Intersalt results has been widely criticized due to the fact that Intersalt was not a longitudinal study (i.e., blood pressure and salt consumption information were not recorded over several decades in specific individuals). Thus, it is a major leap to suggest that salt consumption may cause blood pressure to increase with age based on the Intersalt findings. For example, if the average blood pressure of seventy year olds today is higher than twenty year olds, it could be that the older group always had higher blood pressure even when they were twenty: this is known as a cohort effect and there is compelling evidence that this may account for the Intersalt findings.[36] Further, even if blood pressure does increase in populations where salt consumption is high, salt intake would be just one of many possible explanations. The societies that were examined by the Intersalt team often differed dramatically in terms of other dietary and lifestyle factors. For these reasons, the age and blood pressure relationship that was reported by the Intersalt investigators has been referred to as meaningless. Additionally, according to Intersalt detractors the sodium and blood pressure escalation with age connection was not one of the original hypotheses put forth by the investigators in pre-study publications describing the study. In other words, the critics felt that the Intersalt investigators had salt suppressive motives and that they did not find the compelling evidence against salt that they had desired. Thus, in desperation Intersalt researchers performed extensive analyses (sometimes called data dredging) until they found something that could be interpreted as damning about salt.[27] Rarely is a study so widely and enthusiastically praised by one group of people and at the same time smeared by many others as has occurred with Intersalt.

The feud concerning the Intersalt study boiled along for quite some time, however, in 1996 the Intersalt investigators fanned the flames once again by publishing Intersalt Revisited. The Intersalt team had reanalyzed their old data, using what many consider to be extremely controversial statistics, and in effect were now saying "oops, our original analyses underestimated the dangers of salt: salt intake predicts high blood pressure much more than was first reported."[55] Suffice it to say that the arguments put forth in this most recent Intersalt installment were viewed with extreme suspicion and skepticism and the study was not well received by much of the research community.[27]

Although the Intersalt group as well as other investigators have reported correlations between average salt intake and blood pressure across populations, few have found relationships between blood pressure of individuals within a population and salt intake. Similarly, people with high blood pressure do not consume more salt than those with normal blood pressure, in fact, it has been reported that hypertensives eat less sodium. These sorts of findings have been problematic for those who endorse salt suppression for everyone.[56] Further, Americans who are rural have slightly higher blood pressure than those residing in the city but there is no evidence that salt intake differs between the two groups. Also, black Americans tend to have essential hypertension more often than white Americans and salt consumption cannot account for the differences.[57] Some salt suppressors have argued that tendencies for some people to retain salt in their bodies more than others may account for essential hypertension. However, there seems to be a snag here also: the idea that individuals with high blood pressure may not consume more salt but instead tend to retain sodium in their bodies has generally not been supported by the best research.

People with essential hypertension do not have more sodium in their bodies than those without high blood pressure.[58]

Summary and Conclusions

The salt debate is a testimony to the lack of objectivity of science in practice. When all else fails some salt scientists call the perceived rival a shameless carpetbagger and resort to the use of complex and controversial statistical procedures and data dredging in an attempt to manipulate their findings to match their preconceptions. It seems that all too often fancy statistics are used to conceal and confuse and interpretations of results are made cockeyed so that they are in harmony with a longstanding agenda. The most obvious example is the Intersalt study but this tendency is also evident in the research coming from some of the salt subverts. Upon reading some of the salt literature one is often left wondering why the journal editors allowed certain studies to be published with such blatant problems.

Although the negative reputation of salt does not yet rival that of the ultimate nutrient villain dietary fat, the salt suppressors are making every attempt possible to push what they perceive to be the undeniable dangers of salt into the consciousness of all Americans. An attempt has been made in this chapter to provide a brief but balanced view of the science surrounding the reputation of salt. Although the health risks and benefits of universal salt reduction should be and certainly are being examined and debated, to the chagrin of some salt suppressors who ardently believe that the available evidence already proves without a doubt that salt is guilty of being a seductive killer, perhaps we should be concerned about how a stronger message directed at reducing salt intake will be assimilated into the consciousness of Americans. What will be the cost in terms of the development of new food fears and how will these newly assimilated ideas impact us nutritionally? In other words if the food industry, our government, and lay media increase the intensity of the message against salt and push it further in the direction of infamy there will likely be some negative repercussions.

Notes

1. M. E. Oakes and C. S. Slotterback, What's in a name? A comparison of men's and women's judgements about food names and their nutrient contents, *Appetite* 36
2. M. E. Oakes and C. S. Slotterback, Judgements of food healthfulness: food name stereotypes in adults over age 25, *Appetite* 37 (2001ᶜ), 1-8.
3. M. E. Oakes and C. S. Slotterback, The good, the bad, and the ugly: Characteristics used by young, middle-aged, and older men and women, dieters and non-dieters to judge the healthfulness of foods, *Appetite* 38 (2002), 91-97.
4. G. A. MacGregor and H. E. de Wardener, *Salt, diet and health* (Cambridge, UK: Cambridge University Press 1998), 100-102.
5. G. R. Kerr and M. Z. Nichaman, Salt and hypertension, *Public Health Review* 14 (1986) 25-104.
6. B. F. Liebman and M. F. Jacobson, Sodium content of restaurant foods in United States are high, *British Medical Journal* 315 (1997), 488.
7. A. M. Pearson and A. M. Wolzak, Salt-its use in animal products-a human health dilemma. *Journal of Animal Science* 54 (1982) 1263-1278.
8. M. F. Jacobson and B. F. Liebman, Sodium in processed foods, *American Journal of Clinical Nutrition* 63 (1996) 138.
9. A. Eisenberg, H. E. Murkoff, and S. E. Hathaway, *What to expect the first year* (New York: Workman Publishing 1996), 137.
10. A. Eisenberg, H. E. Murkoff, and S. E. Hathaway, What to expect the first year (New York: Workman Publishing 1996), 391.
11. S. Tisdale, *Lot's wife: Salt and the human condition* (New York: Henry Holt and Company 1988).
12. B.F. Liebman, High blood pressure: The end of an epidemic? *Nutrition Action Health Letter* 27 (2000).
13. G. A. MacGregor and H. E. de Wardener, *Salt, diet and health.*
14. G. R. Kerr and M. Z. Nichaman, Salt and hypertension, 34.
15. G. A. MacGregor and H. E. de Wardener, *Salt, diet and health,* 83-87.
16. H. Levenstein, *Revolution at the table* (New York: Oxford University Press 1988), 86-90.
17. V. Herbert and S. Barrett, *Vitamins and "health" foods: The great American hustle* (Philadelphia, PA: George F. Stickley Company 1981), 88.
18. D. Armstrong and E. M. Armstrong, *The great American medicine show* (New York: Prentice Hall 1991), 127.
19. R. S. Berghoff and A. S. Geraci, The influence of sodium chloride on blood pressure, *The Illinois Medical Journal* 56 (1929) 395-397.
20. C. B. Chapman and T. B. Gibbons, The diet and hypertension, *Medicine* 29 (1949) 29-69.
21. C. B. Chapman and T. B. Gibbons, The diet and hypertension, 43.
22. C. B. Chapman and T. B. Gibbons, The diet and hypertension, 44-45.
23. G. R. Kerr and M. Z. Nichaman, Salt and hypertension, 69.
24. C. B. Chapman and T. B. Gibbons, The diet and hypertension, 46.
25. G. A. MacGregor and H. E. de Wardener, *Salt, diet and health,* 89.
26. P. P. Stein and H. R. Black, The role of diet in the genesis and treatment of hypertension, *Clinical Nutrition* 77 (1993) 831-847.
27. G. Taubes, The (political) science of salt, *Science* 281 (August 1998), 898-907.
28. L. J. Appel, et al., A Clinical trial of the effects of dietary patterns on blood pressure, *The New England Journal of Medicine* 336 (1997), 1117-1124.

29. F. M. Sacks, et al., Effects on blood pressure of reduced dietary sodium and the dietary approaches to stop hypertension (DASH) diet, *The New England Journal of Medicine* 344 (2001), 3-10.
30. G. Taubes, A DASH of data in the salt debate, *Science* 288 (2000) 1319.
31. D. A. Freedman and D. B. Petitti, Salt and blood pressure conventional wisdom reconsidered, *Evaluation Review* 25 (2001), 267-287.
32. L. H. Kuller, Salt and blood pressure, American Journal of Hypertension 10 (1997) 29S-36S.
33. G. Watt and J. T. Hart, Slow decremental change in dietary sodium load in whole population is needed, *British Medical Journal* 315 (1997), 486.
34. G. A. MacGregor and H. E. de Wardener, *Salt, diet and health*, 193-196.
35. D. Riccardella and J. Dwyer, Salt substitutes and medicinal potassium sources: Risks and benefits, *The American Dietetic Association* 85 (1985), 471-474.
36. N. Graudal and A. Galloe, Should dietary salt restriction be a basic component of antihypertensive therapy, *Cardiovascular Drugs and Therapy* 14 (2000), 381-386.
37. F. C. Luft, C. D. Morris, and M. H. Weinberger, Compliance to a low-salt diet, *American Journal of Clinical Nutrition* 65 (1997), 698S-703S.
38. G. A. MacGregor and H. E. de Wardener, *Salt, diet and health*, 175-191.
39. T. Antonios and G. MacGregor, Salt more adverse effects, *Lancet* 348 (1996), 250-251.
40. M. H. Alderman et al, Scientists' statement regarding data on the sodium-hypertension relationship and sodium health claims on food labeling, *Nutritional Reviews* 55 (1997) 172-175.
41. G. R. Kerr and M. Z. Nichaman, Salt and hypertension, 44-51.
42. D. Labarthe and C. Ayala, Nondrug interventions in hypertension prevention and control, *Cardiology Clinics* 20 (2002) 249-263.
43. L. J. Beilin, Lifestyle and hypertension—an overview, *Clinical and experimental hypertension* 21 (1999) 749-762.
44. H. E. de Wardener and N. M. Kaplan, On the assertion that a moderate restriction of sodium intake may have adverse health effects, *American Journal of Hypertension* 6 (1993) 810-814.
45. G. R. Kerr and M. Z. Nichaman, Salt and hypertension, 75.
46. I. Bou-Holaigah, P. C. Rowe, J. Kan, and H. Calkins, The relationship between neurally mediated hypotension and the chronic fatigue syndrome, *JAMA* 274 (1995), 961-967.
47. M. H. Alderman, H. Cohen, and S. Madhavan, Dietary sodium intake and mortality: the National Health and Nutrition Examination Survey (NHANES 1), *Lancet* 351 (1998), 781-785.
48. T. C. Beard, A salt-hypertension hypothesis, *Journal of Cardiovascular Pharmacology* 16 (1990), S35-S38.
49. G. R. Kerr and M. Z. Nichaman, Salt and hypertension, 73.
50. G. R. Kerr and M. Z. Nichaman, Salt and hypertension, 44-45.
51. G. A. MacGregor and H. E. de Wardener, *Salt, diet and health*, 127-135.
52. G. A. MacGregor and H. E. de Wardener, *Salt, diet and health*, 89-90.
53. G. A. MacGregor and H. E. de Wardener, *Salt, diet and health*, 122-124.
54. J. E. Dimsdale, Stalked by the past: The influence of ethnicity on health, *Psychosomatic Medicine* 62 (2000), 161-170.
55. P. Elliott, et al., Intersalt revisited: further analyses of 24 hour sodium excretion and blood pressure within and across populations, *British Medical Journal* 312 (1996), 1249-1253.

56. G. R. Kerr and M. Z. Nichaman, Salt and hypertension, 66-68.

57. G. R. Kerr and M. Z. Nichaman, Salt and hypertension, 38.

58. J. D. Swales, Salt and high blood pressure: A study in education, persuasion, and naivete. In D. Anderson, ed.: *A diet of reason: Sense and nonsense in the healthy eating debate* (Social Affairs Unit 1986).

5

Sowing Sugar's Bitter Harvest

To a nutritional scientist the word "sugar" has a broader meaning than it does for most lay people. All sugars are carbohydrates some of which are very simple and are termed monosaccharides (single sugars). The monosaccharides are naturally abundant in many fruits and vegetables with glucose (also called dextrose) and fructose being the most common types. Galactose is a simple sugar that is found in dairy foods. The white granules that we use in baking and pour or spoon into our beverages and onto cereal are slightly more complex than these simple sugars and go by the name sucrose. Sucrose is a disaccharide (double sugar) consisting of the two single sugars, glucose and fructose, joined together. Lactose or milk sugar is also a disaccharide and is composed of the simple sugar glucose joined with galactose. Edible fruits are particularly rich in mono- and disaccharides, for example, 86 percent of the dry weight of an apple is sugar. The United States Food and Drug Administration which regulates food labeling defines the term "sugars" that we see on food labels as the total grams of mono- and disaccharides in a serving of the food. Also, the *Dietary Guidelines* coming from our United States Department of Agriculture advises us to "choose beverages and foods to moderate sugars." Thus, although sucrose (table sugar) likely has a more negative reputation than other types of sugars (e.g., fructose) among some Americans, our federal government apparently does not consider the various sugars distinct in terms of health value.[1]

More complex carbohydrates contain many sugar units bonded together and are referred to as polysaccharides (many sugars). Polysaccharides, contrary to the more simple sugars, are elements of our foods that generally have a very good reputation these days: they include the complex carbohydrates (i.e., starches), which mainstream nutrition experts advise us to eat in large quantities, and are components of fiber which is also highly praised by modern nutrition authorities. Ironically, given the varying reputations of different carbohydrates, all carbohydrates (with the exception of fiber) are reduced to the simple sugar glucose (blood sugar) in humans through the process of digestion, and when pure, carbohydrates do not contain vitamins and minerals. Finally, different than fat, protein, vitamins, and minerals, carbohydrates are not required for our survival.[2]

As already described what we call white or table sugar is one of several chemicals of the carbohydrate family, it is found in varying amounts in all fruits and vegetables (fruits have more than vegetables), and is referred to by scientists as sucrose. Although sucrose can be found in all green plants, the most important sources of sucrose for human consumption are sugar cane grass and sugar beet plants.[3] Most of the sucrose that we eat nowadays comes to us in processed foods. Sucrose serves many purposes in processed foods in addition to its contribution as a sweetener. Sucrose, when used in non-yeast raised baked goods, provides a desirable texture, flavor, and color. Additionally, for yeast-raised foods sucrose serves as sustenance for the microorganisms that we call yeast during the fermentation process and inhibits staleness in bread which lengthens shelf life Sucrose affects the freezing point and flavor of ice cream and when used in small amounts acts as a seasoning or spice in cottage cheese. For soft drinks it provides desirable sweetness, enhances flavor, and provides desirable "body" and mouth feel to the beverage (without sucrose people perceive soft drinks to be too watery). For canned goods sucrose blends well with the natural flavors of fruits and vegetables and protects flavors better than alternative sweeteners that may become undesirably bitter or sour with prolonged storage. Additionally, it protects color, freshness, shelf life, and reduces the acidity of canned foods. For processed meats sucrose diminishes the harshness of salt, contributes desirable flavoring, and inhibits the development of harmful bacteria.[4] Finally, in deep-fried foods that are coated in batter sucrose is used in the batter to promote caramelization (i.e., to brown and seal the food inside the batter). Thus, sucrose has many functions in addition to its capacity to promote sweetness, in fact, in many

cases the sweetness that sucrose provides is irrelevant and sometimes even undesirable to food processors.[5]

Confectionary Confusion

Paradoxically, we commonly receive advice from nutritional
authorities and the government reminding us to reduce sugar consumption, however, certain foods that are often recommended in
abundance and which have very good reputations have high contents of various sugars. For example, many fruits (particularly those
that have been dried somewhat) have higher percentages of sugars
(i.e., mono- and disaccharides) than desserts like cake and ice cream.
Certainly, a response from nutritional authorities and the federal
government would be that fruits and vegetables provide us with
many more vitamins and minerals than dessert foods. However,
this is sometimes not the case, for example, a medium apple (a
very reputable food) has over twice the amount of sugars as a cake
donut (a disreputable food) but apples do not have an advantage
over donuts in terms of vitamin and mineral contents (sodium which
is higher in the donut was not included). Fat content is also higher
in the donut but 83 percent of the fat is unsaturated.[6] Donuts also
contain more refined starches but most people do not consider refined starches a negative characteristic when judging food healthfulness: for example, starchy foods like pasta and bagels are
considered very healthful by Americans. One potentially harmful
message that has been incorporated into our thoughts regarding
foods is that the sugars in apples are good for health but that the
sugars found in donuts are bad for us.

The terms "added sugars, " "extrinsic sugars, " and "hidden sugars" were often encountered in the sugar literature. The use of the
term "hidden sugars" was common in less scientific sources by
anti-sugar enthusiasts who emphasized that processors were dis-
guising sugars (often in foods that do not even taste sweet) by
using what they considered to be a variety of deceptive names
(e.g., terms like glucose and dextrose) when listing the ingredients
of the foods. However, now that the total grams of all monosaccharides and disaccharides in a food serving are encompassed in the
nutritional facts panel on the food package under the moniker "sugars, " deception is more difficult. The terms "extrinsic sugars" (which
was encountered primarily in literature from Great Britain) and

"added sugars" (which is more commonly used here in the United States) refer to sugars added during processing or home preparation. We are constantly told by nutrition authorities as well as our own government that we eat too much added sugars but not enough sugary fruits and vegetables. Many sources (particularly older ones) indicate that extrinsic sugars (those that have been added and are not found naturally in foods) are absorbed into the blood faster after ingestion than intrinsic sugars (i.e., those found naturally in fruits and vegetables).[7] Nowadays, contrary to one hundred yours ago, rapid absorption of food is thought to be a negative unhealthful characteristic of food. However, the most recent information on this subject (as will be described a bit later) indicates that extrinsic sugars are often not absorbed more rapidly than intrinsic sugars.[8] Once again, it is easy to assimilate the message that sugar in one type of food is good but in another is bad, however, a viable scientific basis for this belief is elusive.

As described in chapter one, other types of sweeteners often have a better reputation in terms of healthfulness among Americans than sucrose. For example, some folks believe honey or maple sugar to be more natural and wholesome alternatives to white granulated sugar. Many purveyors of nutritional information have advised Americans to substitute honey for sugar,[9] apparently not realizing that honey is primarily sugar. Honey has no meaningful advantage over sucrose in terms of vitamin and mineral or sugar content, however, honey does have more calories than sucrose. The sugars in honey are mostly of the monosaccharide type with no known health advantage over pure sucrose. Honey sugars are mostly fructose (35-40 percent) and glucose (30-35 percent) with a little sucrose and maltose (the latter two both being disaccharides). Maple sugar has more minerals than pure sucrose but is mostly sucrose itself with some traces of other sugars (e.g., glucose and fructose). Another substitute is high fructose corn syrup (HFCS), which is now used particularly in the beverage industry (e.g., soft drinks) but also in many other processed foods (e.g., cereals, baked goods, dairy foods, and candy). Corn sweeteners are derived from cornstarch which is then converted to corn syrup (almost all of which is glucose) then further processed into a sugary concoction with a chemical structure similar to sucrose. There is no evidence that corn sweeteners are more healthful than sucrose and although called high fructose this sweetener has no more fructose than ordinary sucrose but is cheaper than sucrose.[10]

Sucrose consumption among Americans has dropped over the past thirty years as our intake of corn sweeteners has escalated. Americans gulp or gobble more caloric sweeteners (e.g., corn sweeteners, sucrose, honey, maple syrup) than ever before, an estimated 150 to 160 pounds per year for every American, [10] compared to about 90 pounds per person in 1910.[11] An estimated 16 percent of our total energy intake now comes in the form of added sugars.[12] There is no recommended daily value for sweeteners, however, the federal government does suggest a six to eighteen teaspoon maximum daily (depending on your total caloric intake) for "added" sweeteners for most Americans (once again the sugars in fruits and vegetables do not count). Thus, we have plenty of room for improvement given that the average American slurps, swigs, or munches an estimated thirty-three teaspoons of added caloric sweeteners per day. Our sweet tooth is satisfied mostly by corn sweeteners rather than sucrose these days and the greatest percentage of added sweeteners is introduced to our bodies as soft drinks.[10] Amazingly, no chewing is necessary for almost half of the added sugars that Americans consume (the figure is over 60 percent for young adult men) for these sugary concoctions are sipped or swilled in the form of beverages.[12]

In the views of many nutritional authorities, our federal government provides unnecessarily vague advice regarding sugars. The federal government's Dietary Guidelines advise us to "choose beverages and foods to moderate your intake of sugar."[1] There may be some merit in the government's approach regarding sugars (i.e. in not advising us to avoid specific foods). Perhaps we should be wary of those who preach that individual foods are either "good" (e.g., an apple) or "bad" (e.g., a potato) for health due to the fact that these recommendations can be so easily distorted by a food's reputation for health which is frequently (as stated before) not in agreement with views on the nutrient contents of the food. Also, there is a significant controversy concerning the health benefits and dangers of nutrients (e.g., as were already described for dietary fat) and stronger statements from our government may not be justified. On the other hand some disgruntled purveyors of nutritional wisdom consider the government's nutritional guidelines ineffective and confusing (some of these guidelines without a doubt are confusing). However, these authorities have never considered the potential impact of food reputations on the dietary recommendations that they provide or that their recommendations may contribute to stereotypical notions about foods. For example, the authorities from Harvard who are advising us to avoid potatoes because compared to other vegetables the spud offers little more than starch[13] are perhaps unknowingly influenced by food reputations and are also contributing to the negative reputation of the potato. Also, some purveyors of nutritional advice often downplay the controversies concerning food nutrients (e.g., like dietary fat), are often adamant in their beliefs that there are "good" and "bad" foods, reject advice suggesting the importance of eating a balanced diet, and perceive that the ambiguity of the government's message regarding, for example, sugar, expresses a greater concern for the economic welfare of the sugar industry rather than the health of Americans.[14] No doubt political and economic issues influence the dietary advice that we receive from the government: one obvious example is for soft drinks. If nutritional issues were the sole basis of government recommendations we would likely receive specific advice to reduce soft drink consumption (rather than moderate intake of sugars). Soft drinks provide no nutrients except calories (which most of us do not need) and when confronted with these facts representatives from the industry make ridiculous statements such as soft drinks give us energy and necessary fluids.

The Sweet Old Days

Contrary to our current views of sugar as being a sort of dietary nuisance, a few hundred years ago sugar generally was viewed much more positively. Sugar had five principal functions in colonial times: as medicine, spice/condiment (when used in small quantities), sweetener (when used in large quantities), preservative, and decorative material.[15] Our forefathers were apt to view sugar as both medicinal (e.g., for treating colds and coughs) and as a highly luxurious treat. George Washington employed his own French candy maker and Thomas Jefferson had a fondness for a certain personally perfected ice cream recipe.[16] In fact, one of the few and apparently minor concerns regarding cane sugar consumption, at least in the Northern states, that existed 200 years ago involved reservations about the use of slave labor in its production. Due partially to the concerns of abolitionists but owing also to the fragility and vulnerability of the sugar cane plant, attempts were made to discover acceptable cane sugar substitutes from sources like corn stalks, pine trees, acorns, chestnut trees, and milk. However, only the sugar beet proved to be a viable alternative source of refined sugar and there was a bonus: sugar beets could be grown in cooler climates.[17]

Due in part to the rapidly increasing use of sugar beets in refined sugar production during the mid to late 1800s, sugar consumption increased dramatically during the nineteenth century. By 1870, it was estimated that the average American ate forty-one pounds of sugar annually, over six times what their ancestors had in the 1790s. By 1901 average yearly consumption was up to sixty-eight pounds per person. Consequently, refined sugar was transformed from its status as a luxury commodity, available only to the wealthy, to a necessity in every household. Less fortunate white Americans and most blacks were forced to settle for the dregs of refined sugar processing, that is, dark and viscous molasses rather than the pure and wholesome white granules. Ironically, as we all know, these days the darkness of foods often connote characteristics such as natural, wholesome, and nutritious, but one hundred years ago many Americans would have considered honey and maple syrup old fashioned, primitive, and nutritionally inferior to white sugar.[18]

Although mainstream Americans viewed sugar positively well into the twentieth century, occasional negative commentaries about products made from the sweetener have been evident for quite some time. For example, in the early nineteenth century a few Americans were concerned about candy consumption in children. Some elite reform-minded writers of this time period expressed fears that candy consumption particularly in misguided and poverty-stricken children would ultimately result in intemperance, gluttony, disease, and debauchery. Some even felt that a childhood sweet tooth if indulged would ultimately in adulthood develop into a craving for alcohol. Thus, not only was candy consumption considered addictive itself, it could also foster the development of drug habits. This may seem ridiculous but the critics had some concrete examples that reinforced this candy-drug connection: some candies came in the shape of liquor bottles with the word "gin" printed on the label and other candies actually had some liqueur concealed in the center. Similarly, as you may expect there were reformers who preached that candy consumption caused children to prematurely adopt adult vices like sexual indulgences and tobacco use (the latter being not so farfetched given the availability of chocolate cigarettes in the late nineteenth century) as well as gambling and stealing. Additionally, there were concerns that confections, particularly children's candies, would ruin teeth and that they were adulterated with harmful ingredients such as toxic dyes, lead, mercury, glue, and even powdered glass (to make them glisten). Further, it was feared that the candy wrappers themselves often left harmful residues. Consequently, in the late nineteenth century, mothers were encouraged to make candy at home for their children. Although these early reformers of sugary fare may have had good intentions, a snobbish theme was often evident: the unpackaged hard candies most available to poor kids were considered dangerous but the same ingredients when wrapped in a fancy package and sold at a higher price were more often viewed as harmless pleasure.[19]

As sugar became more abundant and inexpensive sweets became more and more associated not only with childish innocence but also with femininity, passion, romance, and weakness. According to sugar historian Wendy Woloson, over the past 200 years we have developed tendencies to view sugary products (aside from sugary medicines) as being most enticing to those perceived to have little impulse control, that is, women and children. Thus, it was thought that women were particularly vulnerable to the addictive and impassioning effects of sweets such as ice cream, chocolate and soda water concoctions. Some reformers were extremely concerned about female indulgence regarding these products.[18]

Interestingly, some writers have suggested the possibility that among the laboring poor it was conventional to give working fathers priority access to the best foods available to the family. Thus, after sugar lost much of its medicinal mystique (i.e., in the nineteenth and twentieth centuries) poor families may have over-relied on sugar to feed their children in order to better ensure that working fathers had the more costly and nutritive protein foods to eat. Essentially, the chilling (and at that time) unspoken meaning was that babies, small children, and maybe to a less extent mothers were considered more expendable and sucrose was used as a sort of "population control." One author made the case that the Reagan administration's attempt a few years ago to define sucrose-rich catsup as a "vegetable" for school lunch programs is a more recent demonstration of our disregard for the health of poor children.[20]

Americans have progressively become more and more fascinated with chocolate over the past 200 years. By the early nineteenth century some Americans were convinced of the restorative, nourishing and energy producing effects of chocolate (particularly if served as a beverage and if milk was an ingredient) for infants, children, the elderly, and those recovering from illness. However, soft, luscious bite-sized chocolates were more often viewed with suspicion and as inappropriate for young people. Detractors considered them dangerous, decadent, sinful and indulgent: to these critics chocolate consumption not only stimulated sexual passion (e.g., masturbation) but also represented sexual acts itself.[18] Interestingly, similar to sexual acts and alcohol consumption solitary indulgence of chocolate (i.e., enjoying the delightful tidbits when not in the company of others) was considered most improper. In fact, sugar's association with chocolate (as well as coffee and tea), according to Paul Rozin, has contributed to the sullied reputation of the sweetener.[21] Women were considered most susceptible to the allure of chocolate as well as the physical and spiritual degradation brought on by chronic bonbon eating. It these warnings were not sufficiently dissuasive there were other alarming messages concerning chocolate candy overindulgence: unrestrained candy eating reportedly promoted deterioration of feminine beauty and even emotional withdrawal symptoms (e.g., depression). Ultimately Milton Hershey and other market savvy chocolate barons realized that the lighter colored and more sweetly flavored milk chocolate was more palatable to children and the addition of milk made this candy less objectionable and even "good" for kids. Thus, to some extent the naughty illicit chocolate was made innocent and nice as well as suitable for the little ones.[18]

Modern Candy Crusades

Although sugar maintained much of its luster in the consciousness of the common people throughout most of the twentieth century, when the technology became available to assess the vitamin and mineral content of foods in the first few decades of the twentieth century and it was consequently discovered that sugar contained virtually none of these coveted nutrients, those in health food circles were quick to bespatter sugar as a contributor to malnutrition as well as tooth decay, diabetes, and obesity. However, in the late 1960s and extending through the mid 1970s a vitriolic assault was launched against the reputation of sugar by both lay crusaders and a small portion of the scientific community.[22] It became common and perhaps even fashionable thirty years or so ago for people from a variety of backgrounds to promote the perceived dangers in terms of negative health consequences of sugar consumption. One event that rattled the foundations of sugar's reputation in the consciousness of Americans and pushed the sweetener toward the precipice of damnation came by way of Robert Choate. Choate was the nutrition reformer who claimed that eating cereal-box cardboard would promote better health than consumption of the sugary treats inside the box. Essentially Choate contended that American children were purposefully programmed by the cereal makers to develop sugar addiction and demand sugary goodies, which invariably were woefully lacking in vitamin and mineral content.[23]

The lay critique of Robert Choate concerning sugar captured the public's attention briefly but Choate's efforts paled in comparison to those of John Yudkin, who became known as sugar's most prominent and tireless scientific critic. Starting back in the 1960s and extending till his death in 1995, John Yudkin from the University of London, England railed about the dangers of sugar. Yudkin freely admitted in his published book from 1972 entitled *Sweet and Dangerous* that his views regarding the dangers of sugar as it related to heart disease were at odds with those of Ancel Keys (the father of fat restriction) and that Keys was critical of his (i.e., Yudkin's) research and condemnation of sugar. Yudkin felt that sugar consumption in a population, rather than fat intake as Keys suggested, better predicted coronary mortality in a country. In addition to causing heart disease, Yudkin considered sugary fare to contribute to a hodgepodge of other health problems such as cancer, gout, liver disease, obesity, decreased longevity (apparently even after accounting for increased cancer and heart disease), nutritional deficiencies, hypoglycemia, mental illness, vision problems, skin problems, indigestion, ulcers, diabetes, and of course rotten teeth. Somewhat different from today's general condemnation concerning all refined carbohydrates, Yudkin stated repeatedly that the health problems associated with eating sucrose often did not generalize to other carbohydrates, for example, enriched white flour. To him sucrose was uniquely dangerous and that any controversy revolving around the health value of white or whole wheat bread was based on misinformation because one was as healthful as the other. Yudkin assumed that sucrose consumption, more so than other carbohydrates, was uniquely dangerous, in part, because it produced rapid and dramatic escalations in blood sugar.[7] We now know that other carbohydrates, even those having a much better reputation among Americans than sugar (e.g., complex carbohydrates), can stimulate more pronounced increases in blood sugar than can table sugar. The term "glycemic index" is often used nowadays when describing a food's potential to cause rapid upward shifts in blood sugar levels. Interestingly, a food's glycemic index can be influenced by many factors, for example, ripeness, the method of preparation, and the other foods or ingredients consumed during the meal. The current wisdom among many authorities is that readily digestible foods that provide a rapid burst of available fuel to our body's tissues are unhealthful. Thus, having a high glycemic index is thought to be a negative characteristic of a food. However, some foods with very positive reputations such as carrots, Cheerios, and wheat bread have a higher glycemic index than does sucrose.[8]

Although Yudkin's review of sugar was scathing, his criticisms of the sweetener appear meager in comparison to those coming from a nonscientific source penned in 1975 and entitled *Sugar Blues*. Although sugar is still widely criticized today, *Sugar Blues* stands out more than any other work before or since in terms of its far-reaching and farfetched attempts to vilify sugar: the author (William Dufty) depicted sugar quite literally as a scourge to humanity. Dufty implicated sucrose as being a contributor to a variety of what are often termed mental illnesses such as schizophrenia, addiction, and alcoholism. Dufty argued that what was perceived as witchcraft several hundred years ago may in fact have been due to a madness brought on by eating sugar. Additionally, a case was made by Dufty for sugar being a possible cause of the bubonic plague (ironically, during the actual epidemic some people considered sugar a remedy for the black death), tuberculosis, suicide, epilepsy, crime, divorce, baldness, impotency, varicose veins, and of course cancer. Sugar was also said to be responsible for all sorts of more minor discomforts of modern life such as diarrhea, constipation, gas, and hemorrhoids. Further, although a precise explanation was not offered (perhaps we can be thankful for that) Dufty conveyed that sugar was responsible for "the need for toilet paper."[24] And, if you should happen to have any discomfort related to the menstrual cycle, well that was likely caused by sugar also. Dufty's tunnel vision regarding sugar was astonishing, he conveyed that smoking cigarettes, except when sugar is used to process the tobacco, is likely helpful for weight reduction and that smoking is more healthful than eating food that contains sugar. Additionally, according to Dufty, if you stop eating sugar you can lie in the sun without protective lotion and not have to worry about burning or skin damage. And lounging in the outdoors will be all the more pleasant because you will not need those smelly bug repellents, mosquitoes will no longer find you appealing once you give up the sweets. Could sugar be responsible for a "significant" number of car accidents? The answer, due to the fact sugar causes "pathological drowsiness and hypoglycemia, " would be a resounding yes according to this sugar critic. Further, in this same treatise some of the more common charges against sugar were also described including of course hypoglycemia (this was thought to cause the drowsiness and mental illness), hyperactivity, vitamin deficiencies (sugar was said to uniquely drain the body of vitamins and minerals), obesity, heart disease, tooth decay, ulcers, and diabetes mellitus.[25] Pictures were provided on the back cover of the book showing Dufty both before and after he became a sugar abstainer. The message appears to be that if you stop eating sugar you will lose any semblance of geekishness, your vision will improve (or at least eye glasses will no longer be necessary), you will become tanned, and look more serious, professional, and fetching to the eye. Although the author attributed all of these astounding health benefits (some of which he experienced himself) to avoiding sugar, he also gave up at least some of his recreational drug habits (both legal and illegal) and started exercising at the same time that he swore off sugar.[26] Dufty attributed his dietary conversion in part to his encounter with the aging film star and food activist Gloria Swanson whom he eventually married (if memory serves, Dufty became Swanson's sixth and final husband).

A year after the publication of Dufty's calumnious volume, came a third book authored by pediatrician Lendon Smith and titled *Improving Your Child's Behavior Chemistry*. Smith became somewhat of a TV personality during the 1970s, he was known as "the children's doctor" through his own TV series and his appearances on popular talk shows (*The Phil Donohue Show*) and even late night TV (*The Tonight Show*). Smith spoke of the dramatic shifts he had observed during his thirty-year tenure as a children's doctor concerning the type of problems that parents presented to him. The increased frequency of problems such as night wakefulness, irritability, aggression, temper tantrums, head aches, stomach pain, and dozens of other bodily complaints were largely due to the toxic effects of addictive sugar on our children's nervous systems (he also had grievances with white bread and milk). Smith presented his thoughts with a pseudoscientific spin: he related that sugar, through its effects on blood sugar, inhibits the parts of our central nervous system responsible for pleasant, rational and civilized behavior and stimulates brain areas responsible for primitive, impulsive, and sinister conduct. More concisely stated, sugar harnesses Dr. Jekyll and unleashes Mr. Hyde or alternatively sugar releases our dark side exposing our more basic and seamy characteristics (the reference to *Star Wars* was mine).[27]

The crusaders against sugar were apparently influential, by the mid-1970s heightened suspicion concerning sugar was evident in consumer interviews. Many interviewees expressed the ideas that sugar could produce a sort of high (especially in kids), sugar can make you fat, and that the sweetener is associated with additives and artificial coloring and flavoring. Additionally, many people had the impression that if a product contained sugar then it could not be nutritious.[28] Finally, these tirades over sugar, which as we shall see were for the most part never supported by the mainstream scientific community and still aren't, spurred expert committees to rush head long in establishing dietary goals for daily sugar intake before anyone actually knew how much sugar the average American consumes in a day. In other words, they placed the cart in front of the horse. In fact, it has been suggested that the established guideline for sugar consumption was set at a level similar to what Americans were already faring at the time. Thus, unbeknownst to the impetuous experts at the time, no adjustment was necessary for the average American.[29]

The Science of Sugar

Although John Yudkin certainly took a scientific approach in his explorations of the dangers of sugar, for better or worse most of the inflammatory claims made by Yudkin and other crusaders against sugar in the 1970s have substantially faded in the consciousness of Americans and never became well established in the scientific community.

Although one eighteenth-century physician considered sucrose a cure-all (with only one downside, it could make women too fat), [30] a controversy remains today regarding the contribution of sugars to obesity. It is generally accepted by food scientists that humans and other mammals have an innate preference for sweet foods. Further and as you may expect, there is research available showing that we will eat sweet foods like ice cream even after filling up on other foods (e.g., sandwiches, chips, and bananas). However, this effect is not specific for sweets, other tasty but non-sugary foods like pizza also stimulated eating in these folks. [31] Surprisingly, some research findings suggest that those who consume lots of caloric sweeteners tend to be leaner than those of us who fare smaller amounts of sugars. Perhaps, as was suggested for dietary fat, healthy energetic people consume more food (including sugars) than the rest of us. [32] Ironically, the folksy wisdom that many of us remember as kids was that sweets tend to spoil our appetites: implying somehow that a little sweet food would fill us up and make other foods less desirable. However, there is no evidence that sweets have a unique ability to satisfy the appetite, in fact, several studies have shown that if people consume 100 calories of sugars they do not fully compensate by eating 100 fewer calories in an ensuing meal. Findings such as these suggest that sweets do not quell our appetites but instead may cause us to overeat. However, there is no evidence that sugars are different from any other carbohydrate in this regard at least for most people. [29] Perhaps it is worth mentioning that there is some evidence that liquid carbohydrates are less likely to quench our appetites than solid carbohydrate foods. Thus, high carbohydrate beverages may contribute to obesity more than similar amounts of energy consumed in solid foods. Certainly it is widely accepted that both soft drink consumption (more than any other food) and obesity have increased among Americans over the past few decades and fat kids tend to drink more soft drinks than leaner children. [10] Astonishingly, per capita soft drink consumption has increased a whopping 500 percent over the past fifty years. [33]

Any reasonably alert person over age thirty can testify to the jumbo sizing of soft drink containers over the past couple of decades. By way of a favorite hobby (i.e., metal detecting), I have developed a more broad perspective of how our beverage habits have changed over the past seventy years or so. While searching for artifacts and coins from our past in old picnic grounds that have been reclaimed by mother nature, I have always been impressed with how small the soda bottles were that I sometimes stumbled upon. Before 1950, six to seven once soda bottles were typical but nowadays of course nothing of this sort is available. The number of milk bottles of all sizes (some as small as half a pint) encountered while metal detecting is also noteworthy; they are from a dozen different dairies in or in close proximity to Scranton, Pennsylvania. Those dairies are gone now and milk consumption has been declining steadily for the past half century in the United States. Obviously our beverage habits have changed dramatically over the past fifty years or so as soda has displaced milk in the diets of American kids and low calcium intake has become a public concern. Perhaps in part due to concerns about dietary fat, the percentage of teenage girls who routinely drink milk has plummeted over the past twenty-five years Additionally, soft drink consumption in children from the United States is associated with reduced intake of not only calcium but also riboflavin, vitamin A, vitamin C, folic acid, and phosphorous.[34]

As described earlier, John Yudkin believed that sucrose caused heart disease but what does our best science suggest about this issue? Starting back in the 1950s it was observed that feeding participants high carbohydrate diets in the form of liquid formulas altered blood lipid levels in a negative fashion (e.g., causing increased amounts of blood triglycerides which predict heart disease). In the ensuing decades some researchers reported that subjects fed staggering amounts of mono- or disaccharide sugars (as much as 85 percent of total energy intake) with little or no dietary fat showed increased blood tryglyceride levels. Such diets of course were not conducive to health and, thus, were of short duration (i.e., a few days). Incidentally, the diets that were found to cause the most extreme adverse reactions in blood lipid levels were of liquid form with little dietary fiber.[35] There is no evidence that sugars in the amounts commonly consumed by Americans today causes adverse changes in blood lipids. The American Heart Association (AHA) is now providing information about the possible dangers of high-carbohydrate-low-fat diets in general. Such diets, according to the AHA, may increase coronary disease risk (e.g., by decreasing HDL cholesterol and increasing triglycerides) in some people as well as promote obesity and malnutrition. The AHA does not, however, suggest that sucrose or any other sugar is disproportionately responsible for such problems compared to complex carbohydrates.[36]

During the heyday of sugar bashing it was frequently claimed that eating sugary foods caused diabetes (i.e., diabetes mellitus). However, there is no evidence that sugars or any other carbohydrates cause diabetes. The mainstream wisdom now is that excessive calorie intake, which as described above may be fostered by consumption of sugary beverages, leads to weight gain and for some of us diabetes. Thus, any connection to sugar intake as it concerns diabetes is indirect, hinging on the capacity of sugary foods and beverages to promote obesity.[10]

Although the concept that eating sugary fare might cause us to behave badly was first documented as early as 1922, it took the faddish fury coming primarily from the lay literature and pseudoscience of the 1970s to bring the idea that sugar consumption caused hyperactivity, aggression, and crime to the public consciousness. Early on, some folks speculated that an allergic response (or food intolerance) to sucrose might be responsible for hyperactivity in children. A second theory implicated sugar indirectly: the idea was based on the premise that sugary foods are inherently low in other nutrients (of course this is not always true) and that consumption of sweets results in malnutrition which causes crime. Others who considered themselves sugar authorities, mostly from fringe medical backgrounds, argued that hypoglycemia caused by "added" and "hidden" sucrose was responsible for behavior problems in children and adults. Although the mainstream science considered it farfetched, the hypothesis that sugar triggered hypoglycemia and misbehavior was panned for all it was worth, for ultimately it was offered as a possible cause of aggression and delinquency. This half-baked hype was exploited by social workers, criminologists, and judges, e.g., changes were made in the diets of those already imprisoned and some courts even mandated that juvenile offenders participate in dietary regimes or go to jail. One probation officer described to the U.S. Senate Select Committee in 1977 how she successfully treated offenders by removing sugar from their diets.[37] And as you may recall, the legal community was eager to reap the benefits of the hyped dangers of sugar as the famed "Twinkie defense" was offered as a legal argument. The idea being that criminals were not responsible for their misdeeds but instead sugar caused diminished capacity and made them commit crimes. One high profile case from 1979 involved an incident where a man climbed through a city hall window (to avoid metal detectors) and subsequently shot and killed the mayor of San Francisco and another city worker. His lawyers claimed that eating unwholesome sugary foods had created a chemical imbalance in the assailant's brain. The attacker was convicted of voluntary manslaughter (rather than a more serious homicide conviction), which set off a public uproar and ultimately led California voters to eliminate the diminished capacity defense. However, make no mistake about it, this hypoglycemic perspective was embraced with some enthusiasm and perhaps relief by portions of the lay public, for example, parents who were desperate to find reasons for perceived misbehaviors in their own children. On the other hand, to the mainstream scientific community this explanation for misbehavior never was sufficient since it was accepted that hypoglycemia was an extremely rare condition. Succinctly stated, the sugar and hyperactivity/attention span connection has been studied extensively over the past few decades and is not at all supported by our best science. Such studies often involve giving a group of children, who are deemed by their parents or teachers as vulnerable to the adverse effects of sucrose, either sucrose or artificial sweetener under blind conditions (i.e., the children, parents and researchers were unaware of who actually received sugar). Under these controlled conditions the vast majority of research shows no increase in activity or inattention even when the individual (i.e., parent or teacher) who considered the child to be sensitive to sugar in the first place was used as the rater, and some investigators have actually reported calming effects in children after sucrose administration.[38] Thus, it is likely not sugar that causes excessive arousal in kids but instead the stimulation associated with the times it is consumed (e.g., trick or treating, birthday parties, holidays gatherings, and sleepovers). Further, the idea that eating sugary foods caused hypoglycemia or nutrient deficiencies and ultimately crime always had weak roots in the scientific community. The studies in support of these perspectives were few, for example, the research suggesting that eating sugary food caused malnutrition and, thus, criminal behavior came primarily from one California-based criminologist. Generally, the research that connects sugar and crime has been described as flawed.[37] For instance, the methods used to measure hypoglycemia in this research were often inaccurate, unreliable, and outright goofy (e.g., hair analysis and numerous paper and pencil tests were used).[39] The "sugar causing crime" message seems to have withered on the vine to some extent from lack of interest and support from rigorous mainstream science.

The idea that sugary fare promotes tooth decay was documented for the first time at least 400 years ago. Of all the afflictions that sugars have been said to promote, the only one that has mainstream scientific acceptance concerns sugars' role in promoting tooth decay and gum disease. Some sources suggest that sucrose is the worst promoter of tooth decay while other sources are less adamant about sucrose deserving primary villain status in this regard. Any carbohydrate that can be fermented by plaque bacteria can promote tooth decay and gum disease and this includes monosaccharide sugars, disaccharide sugars, and at least some complex carbohydrates. Some experts suggest that the frequency with which we eat fermentable carbohydrates is likely more important than the amount consumed of any single carbohydrate. Thus, lots of snacking is probably not good for our teeth, however, this would depend on what you are snacking. There is some evidence that certain cheeses may actually inhibit tooth decay.[40] Further, as stated earlier, there is no reason to explain why sugars in apples are considered wholesome while sugars in donuts are thought of as poison, however, the texture of some types of fruit flesh and perhaps other ingredients in the fruit may buffer the negative action of fruit and vegetable sugars on tooth and gum disease.

Sugar Advertising

Sugary foods and beverages are often promoted as being fresh, wholesome, crisp, invigorating, refreshing, and vibrant.[41] Additionally, these days it seems that advertisers take advantage of any existing connection or if possible create new connections between their products and sexual imagery and candy is not excluded. One recent impassioning magazine advertisement for candy bars created some steamy imagery by referring to the product's "naked center" and seductively proclaimed "You don't unwrap it, You Undress it" and finally there is a reference to women's underthings with the enticing confession that this most delightful and luscious indulgence is available "without any tricky hooks in the back." Another candy manufacture erotically described one of their products as "The Tunnel of Love."[42] Last month Hershey Foods expressed plans to launch an advertising campaign emphasizing and extolling the seductive, passion-inspiring, and emotionally restorative themes of chocolate's bygone days. One Hershey spokesperson conveyed a desire to resurrect the appeal of chocolate as being both "sexy" and a "magic elixir." Proposed slogans are "available without a prescription, " "resistance is futile, " and "legal in all fifty states."[43] In recent years even foods that are reputedly healthy and wholesome are sometimes advertised with a generous helping of sex appeal. For example, a humorous TV commercial advertising yogurt congers up images of illicit amour by presenting what first appears to be a lovely French-speaking maid who is seated on a balding middle-aged man's lap as she daintily and seductively spoon feeds him yogurt. However, we soon discover, maybe with a little disappointment, as their preadolescent daughter enters the room, that this is not a secret liaison but instead a playful husband and wife. As we all know, sex is commonly used to promote all sorts of things from cars, blue jeans, and mattresses to tobacco, diet foods, weight loss propaganda, and mammograms, however, believe it or not, it is not clear how helpful sex appeal is in advertising. Sex in advertising tends to attract our attention but often does not improve our recall of information provided or even our attitude toward the brand but of course this depends on the gender of the model and the viewer.[44]

Sweet Morality

As has been described, it seems that we have a long and colorful tradition in America of classifying sweet foods or perhaps any food that is particularly pleasing to the palate as immoral and unhealthy. This tradition in combination with other ingredients like reports of the hazards of sugar (often of an outrageous nature) along with sugar's reputation for promoting fatness (when coupled with our more recently developed preferences for slender female bodies) has contributed to the present day view of sugar as a dietary villain particularly for women.[21] For example, although sucrose and other sugars are present in foods that have very good reputations (e.g., fruits and vegetables) some Americans view sugar as toxic even when in trace amounts.[21, 45] According to Paul Rozin and other students of sugar, Americans (and those from Canada and Europe as well) have a strong tendency to believe that if we eat "good" foods and avoid "bad" foods like sugar we become morally and physically (i.e., more slender, attractive, healthy, and long-lived) unique and superior to others.[46] As many of us are aware nowadays, when a fellow American conveys, "I'm trying to be good today" it often does not mean that they are singing hymns or promoting humanitarian efforts or world peace but rather he/she is making an effort to eat reputable foods (e.g., carrots and skim milk). Once again the belief that we are what we eat is evident: if we eat something offensive, we then become offensive.[21] Additionally, sweet foods are often described in terms of morality, for example, angel food and devil's food and recipes for sweet concoctions often include the word "sin" in the names that they go by. This tendency was observed most often for those recipes containing chocolate, for example, "four sins cake" (containing Oreo's, ice cream, chocolate, and cool whip), "chocolate sin cake, " and "the ultimate sin chocolate cake." Perhaps it is ironic (or maybe not) that some of the foods that are considered most infamous in terms of being unhealthful, promoters of obesity, and virtuous to avoid are often the ones we confess to "craving" most, and this is especially true for women.[47] Although our understanding of the concept of "food craving" and the potential causes of cravings (e.g., genetic or social) are not well established, more women admit having food cravings than men, and women more often experience guilt about indulging their cravings. Women acknowledge craving sweet foods (i.e., chocolate, ice cream, and desserts) much more than any other type of food and are much more likely than men to reveal a craving for these sorts of sweetly naughty indulgences. Salty foods (i.e., chips, pretzels, and popcorn) are also craved by women but much less so than sweets.[48]

Summary and Conclusion

Given sugar's reputation in the eyes of most Americans as a contributor to so many health problems, the lack of rigorous scientific evidence pointing to the contribution of sugars in the etiology of disease and misbehavior is astonishing. With the exception of

John Yudkin, the condemnation of sugars came almost exclusively from lay crusaders and pseudoscientists, and none of the vilifications of sugars (aside from their role in tooth decay) is supported by mainstream science. Thus, many ideas about sweets that have become extremely engrained into the average American's consciousness and accepted as nutritional facts first originated and have been disseminated by people that are not most qualified to make dietary recommendations. Additionally, it seems that some people with backgrounds in nutrition or other areas of science (and who should know better) are too willing to accept and peddle this half-baked information concerning sugars.

It seems clear that Americans have assimilated the idea that if a food tastes sweet or contains sugars and is not a raw or recently cooked fruit or vegetable then it must be junk food. The idea appears to be, among many of us, that vitamins and minerals and sugars cannot exist together in the same food. For example, college students rated apples as extremely healthful but caramel apples were not considered nearly as wholesome by those same students Thus, we tend to believe that sweet foods lack vitamins, minerals, protein, and other highly praised nutrients, promote disease, and cause us to gain unwanted pounds. Any evidence suggesting that sugary foods cause disease or obesity is controversial at best and clearly some sweet foods (including those classified as candy) contain reputable nutrients. It was necessary to search no further than a favorite candy bar to find an example: a Snickers bar has significant amounts of five or six vitamins and minerals, almost ten percent of the recommended daily value for protein, and about six percent of recommended fiber. In terms of the amounts of nutrients with positive reputations (e.g., vitamins and minerals) a Snickers bar has a better nutrient profile than many fruits and vegetables but of course most Americans would likely assume otherwise.

Notes

1. US Department of Agriculture, Center for Nutrition Policy and Promotion. Home and Garden Bulletin Number 252. The Food Guide Pyramid. *http://www.usda.gov/cnpp/ Pubs/*Pyramid/fdgdpyr1.pdf. Accessed: October 16, 2002.
2. A. Davidson, *The Oxford companion to food* (Oxford: Oxford University of Press 1999).
3. S. W. Mintz, *Sweetness and power: The place of sugar in modern history* (New York: Viking 1985), 19.

4.   A. Lachmann, The role of sucrose in foods: A comprehensive review of thirty years of research by the international sugar research foundation (The International Sugar Research Foundation, Inc. 1975).
5.   S. W. Mintz, *Sweetness and power:* 206.
6.   J. A. T. Pennington, *Bowes and Church's Food values of portions commonly used* (Philadelphia, PA: Lippincott 1998).
7.   J. Yudkin, *Sweet and dangerous* (New York: Peter H. Wyden, Inc. 1972).
8.   S. B. Roberts, High-glycemic index foods, hunger, and obesity: is there a connection? *Nutritional Reviews* 58 (2000) 163-169.
9.   E. L. Rose, Nutrition: Hidden sugars, Florida Dental Journal 53 (1982) 43.
10. A. M. Coulston and R. K. Johnson, Sugar and sugars: Myths and realities, *Journal of The American Dietetic Association* 102 (2002) 351-353.
11. S. Gerrior and L. Bente, Nutritional content of the U.S. food supply , 1909-99: A summary report. US. Department of Agriculture, Center for Nutrition Policy and Promotion. Home Economics Research Report No. 55.
12. J. F. Guthrie and J. F. Morton, Food sources of added sweeteners in the diets of Americans, *Journal of The American Dietetic Association* 100 (2000) 43-49.
13. W. C. Willett, M. J. Stampfer, Rebuilding the food pyramid, *Scientific American* (January 2003), 64-71.
14. M. Nestle, *Food politics: How the food industry influences nutrition and health* (Berkeley: University of California Press 2002).
15. S. W. Mintz, *Sweetness and power:* 78.
16. W. A. Woloson, *Refined tastes: Sugar, confectionery, and consumers in nineteenth-century America* (Baltimore: The Johns Hopkins University Press 2002), 2.
17. W. A. Woloson, *Refined tastes:* 25-30.
18. W. A. Woloson, *Refined taste.*
19. W. A. Woloson, *Refined tastes: 33-65.*
20. S. W. Mintz, *Sweetness and power:* 149.
21. P. Rozin, Attitudes toward sugar and sweetness in historical and social perspective. In J. Dobbing, ed: *Sweetness* (New York: Springer-Verlag 1986).
22. H. Levenstein, *Paradox of plenty: A social history of eating in modern America* (New York: Oxford University Press 1993), 190-191.
23. J. Rosenthal, Hunger expert says many dry cereals are not nutritious, *New York Times* (Friday, July 24, 1970) 1.
24. W. Dufty, *Sugar Blues* (New York: Warner Book 1975) p. 183
25. W. Dufty, *Sugar Blues* (New York: Warner Book 1975)
26. W. Bennett, The taste that failed, *American Health* July/August (1983).
27. E. W. Mechling and J. Mechling, Sweet talk: The moral rhetoric against sugar, *Central States Speech Journal* 34 (1983) 19-32.
28. C. Fischler, Attitudes toward sugar and sweetness in historical and social perspective. In J. Dobbing, ed: *Sweetness* (New York: Springer-Verlag 1986).
29. H. G. Anderson, Sugars, sweetness, and food intake, *The American Journal of Clinical Nutrition* 62 (1995) 195S.
30. S. W. Mintz, *Sweetness and power:* 106.
31. C. E. Cornell, J. Rodin, and H. Weingarten, Stimulus-induced eating when satiated, *Physiology and Behavior* 45 (1989) 695-704.
32. S. A. Gibson, Are high-fat, high-sugar foods and diets conducive to obesity, *International Journal of Food Sciences and Nutrition* 47 (1996) 405-415.
33. D. S. Ludwig, K. E. Peterson, and S. L. Gortmaker, Relation between consumption of sugar-sweetened drinks and childhood obesity: a prospective, observational analysis. *The Lancet* 357 (2001) 505-508.

34. L. Harnack, J. Stang, and M. Story, Soft drink consumption among US children and adolescents: nutritional consequences, *Journal of The American Dietetic Association* 99 (1999) 436-441.

35. E. J. Parks and M. K. Hellerstein, Carbohydrate-induced hypertriacylglycerolemia: Historical perspective and review of biological mechanisms, *American Journal of Clinical Nutrition* 71 (2000) 412-433.

36. R. M. Krauss, et al. AHA dietary guidelines revision 2000: A statement for healthcare professionals from the nutrition committee of the American Hear Association, *Circulation* 102 (2000) 2284-2299.

37. V. Markes, Exploding the myths about sugar: The case of hypoglycemia. In D. Anderson, ed.: *A diet of reason: Sense and nonsense in the healthy eating debate* (Social Affairs Unit 1986).

38. W. J. White and M. Wolraich, Effects of sugar on behavior and mental performance, *The American Journal of Clinical Nutrition* 62 (1995) 242S.

39. W. E. Doraz, Diet and delinquency: The grounding of four leading theories in human physiology and sociology. In W. B. Essman, ed.: *Nutrients and brain function* (New York: Karger 1987).

40. C. F. Schachtele, Changing perspectives on the role of diet in dental caries formation, *Nutrition News* 45 (1982).

41. S. W. Mintz, *Sweetness and power:* 208.

42. W. A. Woloson, *Refined tastes:* 230-231.

43. S. Elliot, New Hershey advertising campaign extols virtues of eating chocolate, *San Francisco Chronicle*, September 25, 2002.

44. M. Y. Jones, A. J. Stanaland, and B. D. Gelb, Beefcake and cheesecake: Insights for advertisers, *Journal of Advertising* XXVII (1998) 33-51.

45. P. Rozin, M. Ashmore, and M. Markwith, Lay American conceptions of nutrition: Dose insentivity, categorical thinking, contagion, and the monotonic mind, *Health Psychology* 15 (1996), 438-447.

46. S. Mintz, Sugar and morality. In A. M. Brandt and P. Rozin, ed: *Morality and health* (New York: Routledge 1997).

47. S. C. Grogan, R. Bell, and M. Conner. Eating sweet snacks: Gender differences in attitudes and behaviour, *Appetite* 28 (1997) 19-31.

48. H. P. Weingarten and D. Elston, Food cravings in a college population, *Appetite* 17 (1991) 167-175.

6

Four of America's Legendary Favorites

Food scholars have acknowledged for quite some time that society assigns status to individual foods as we do people and that an individual food's status is based on "texture, flavor, rarity, cost, and association" of the food[1] and the individual's social aspirations.[2] Additionally, although many authorities promote the idea that individual foods should not be judged as healthful or unhealthful—only the total diet is important—for better or worse adult Americans of all ages can easily classify individual foods based on their perceived health value.[3] Many purveyors of nutrition information (whether they are legitimate and truly knowledgeable or not) foster this approach to food by praising some foods and criticizing others.

An Apple a Day

Americans perceive the apple to be an extremely healthful food primarily because it is considered to have an abundance of many vitamins and minerals. On the other hand, compared to the name "apple," the nutrient description for the apple was rated much lower in terms of healthfulness by college students and more mature adults.[4, 5] The name "apple" was rated second in terms of healthfulness of the thirty-three foods investigated while the nutrient description for the apple was rated eighth.[4] Do apples in fact have an abundance of many vitamins and minerals? According to *Bowes and Church's Food Values of Portions Commonly Used* by Jean Pennington[6] a medium apple possesses the following percentages of vitamins and minerals (expressed as percentage of the daily value): vitamin A 1 percent, vitamin C 13 percent, vitamin B-1 1 percent, vitamin B-2 1 percent, niacin 5 percent, vitamin B-6 4 percent, vitamin B-12 0 percent, folic acid 1 percent, pantothenic acid 1 percent, potassium 5 percent, calcium 1 percent, phosphorus 1 percent, magnesium 2 percent, iron 1 percent, zinc 0 percent, copper 3 percent, manganese 3 percent. The mineral selenium and vitamins D, E, and K are not provided in Pennington's primary nutrient table, however, none of these reach 10 percent of the daily value in an apple. Thus, a medium apple has only one vitamin (vitamin C) and no minerals that reach or surpass 10 percent of the daily value. Given that the apple does not have the high levels of vitamins and minerals that many Americans suppose, what other factors might explain this fruit's positive reputation in our society?

Although not natural to North America, no other fruit or vegetable approaches the legendary status of the apple in American food history. A recent article in Smithsonian magazine is a testimony to this.[7] In terms of the frequency of reference in stories, poems, fables, myths, and religious books apples are unparalleled. For example, many of us remember hearing as kids the picturesque tale of the legendary American folk hero, Johnny Appleseed, who according to stories, songs, and even a short film which was a favorite for grade school children in the 1960s and 70s, traveled the Midwest planting apple trees. Surprisingly, much of the legend is apparently true. Johnny Appleseed (John Chapman) was born in Massachusetts around 1774, died in about 1845, and in the meantime developed into a genuine American pioneer. Legend has it that his apparel was primitive but arguably practical (most sources say much of this is fact) he allegedly wore a shirt made from a cloth sack, often made his way barefooted (or wore rags for shoes), and a tin cooking pot for a hat. Johnny collected apple seeds from cider mills in Pennsylvania and planted apple tree seedlings throughout the Midwest for almost fifty years but became known to his frontier neighbors for more than just fruit husbandry. For instance, he developed a reputation as a local military hero (e.g., he often warned American settlers of approaching danger during the war of 1812), medicine man, and religious enthusiast. He accepted almost any form of payment for his seeds and sprouts and was apparently eager to offer a generous helping of religious sermon (if given the opportunity) along with his fruit-business dealings to the local settlers.[8, 9]

Although the origins are often pre-American, the health and medicinal virtues of eating apples are firmly grounded in American folklore. According to legend, eating apples daily would maintain health, reduce doctor visits, and cause financial hardships for one's physician. One proverb going back at least to the nineteenth century and possibly of Welsh origin quipped "eat an apple going to bed, make the doctor beg his bread."[10] Then of course there is the more familiar chestnut which first appeared in the United States no more than 100 hundred years ago and which is likely a derivative of the above-mentioned adage "an apple a day keeps the doctor away."[11] An early example of a document extolling the economic, healthful, and medicinal advantages bestowed by eating apples came from a magazine article published in the mid nineteenth century and is provided below. In the article the authors describe apples as being a most adored and wholesome fare and expressed the time-honored lore that daily apple consumption will promote health and reduce encounters with doctors. More specifically, apple consumption was thought to prevent constipation and other gastrointestinal woes as well as ward off fevers. Also, there is a reference to the health benefits of easily digestible foods for which apples were given high marks.

> There is scarcely an article of vegetable food more widely useful and more universally loved than the apple. Why every farmer in the nation has not an apple-orchard where the trees will grow at all, is one of the mysteries. Let every family lay in from two to ten or more barrels, and it will be to them the most economic investment in the whole range of culinaries. A raw mellow apple is digested in an hour and a half, while boiled cabbage requires five hours. The most healthful dessert which can be placed on the table, is the baked apple. If taken freely at breakfast with coarse bread and butter, without meat or flesh of any kind, it has an admirable effect on the general system, often removing constipation, correcting acidities, and cooling of febrile conditions, more effectually than most approved medicines. If families could be induced to substitute the apple, sound, ripe, and luscious, for the pies, cakes, candies, and other sweetmeats with which their children are too often indiscreetly stuffed, there would be a diminution in the sum total of doctors' bills in a single year, sufficient to lay in stock of this delicious fruit for a whole season's use.[12]

As the nineteenth century came to an end apples were still receiving unreserved praise. The following excerpt from an article published in 1896 and entitled "How to Prolong Life" is a testament to this fact.

> The apple is such a common fruit that few persons are familiar with its remarkably efficacious medicinal properties. Everybody ought to know that the very best thing they can do is to eat apples just before going to bed. The apple is excellent brain food because it has more phosphoric acid, in an easily digestible shape, than any other

fruit known. It excites the action of the liver, promotes sound and healthy sleep, and thoroughly disinfects the mouth. It also agglutinates the surplus acids of the stomach, helps the kidney secretions, and prevents calculus growth, while it obviates indigestion and is one of the best preventives of diseases of the throat. Next to lemon and orange it is also the best antidote for the thirst and craving of persons addicted to the alcohol and opium habit.[13]

A few decades later and after the discovery of vitamins, nutrition authorities continued to embrace daily apple consumption as a means to reduce the likelihood of illness and disease and increase energy levels. Further, the apple was praised for having an abundance of vitamins.[14] Also, at this time there was a widely held view that a diet of raw apples was an effective treatment for digestive system woes such as diarrhea, dysentery, and colitis in children.[15] Finally, although the chemist and notable nutrition researcher Elmer Verner McCollum did not classify raw fruits as one of the highly desirable "protective foods" in 1918, by 1930s some purveyors of nutritional information were referring to raw fruits as "highly protective foods."[16]

Some food faddists fed off the wholesome reputation of apples and if anything added to the apple's reputation with their own outlandish claims concerning apples (or apple products). For example, one so-called health expert claimed that downing a mixture of honey and apple cider vinegar would promote good health. However, the FDA disagreed and ultimately removed the concoction (called "Honegar") from the market.[17] Others huckstered the notion that drinking apple juice (not raw apples or cider) could treat ulcers, high blood pressure, or any other health problem.[18] Pseudo-nutritionist Gaylord Hauser promoted something called the "Swiss apple diet that lowers blood pressure and reduces inches."[19]

Reservations concerning eating apples are uncommon in the literature, although Elmer McCollum did convey that "unripe apples and other unripe fruits are unsafe to eat."[20] There were warnings about raw fruits and vegetables in the mid nineteenth century as being vessels for disease transmission (e.g., cholera).[21] During the 1930s, some reform- minded nutrition authorities were critical of American apples because they along with other fruits and vegetables were often sprayed with dangerous chemicals. For example, some warned of the harmful effects of lead arsenate, a common pesticide used on fruits and vegetables. Both components of this compound (i.e., lead and arsenic) were known poisons and were thought to be responsible for a variety of human health problems (skin diseases, listlessness, and retardation).[22] Frederick Schlink expressed disgust concerning the fact that apples had been changed into "factory products"[23] and were "little but sugar water and bulk"[24] produced "with belt-line production techniques."[25] Further, and counter to the ideas expressed by others, Schlink ridiculed the apple, suggesting it was a cause of gastrointestinal woes[26] and despised dried apples as well as other dried fruits because they were treated with the preservative sulphur dioxide gas.[27]

However, to put these criticisms in context, Schlink was writing during an era of heightened anxieties about food additives and adulterants (i.e., 1930s). His muckraking volumes (his own and the one he coauthored with Arthur Kallet) bashed not only apples but also other foods that were generally praised by mainstream nutritional scientists of the day. For example, Schlink considered milk inappropriate for adults, citrus fruits a needless fad, and raw fruits and vegetables of any type to be wholesome only for four-legged critters. Additionally, Schlink comes across to the reader as being a bit of a curmudgeon with a disdain for all new-fangled food innovations. He vituperates to such an extent in this work that the reader feels somewhat dressed down after perusing a few passages.[26]

Thus, why is the apple so highly revered in our society (compared to other foods) and rated as much more healthful than its nutrient description despite its unimpressive nutrient profile? America's ideas about the apple's extreme wholesomeness are a legacy of our distant past (i.e., before the advent of vitamins). Additionally, perhaps the high regard for characteristics such as naturalness, freshness, and absence of fat, which developed mostly in the twentieth century, has somehow compensated for the apple's shortcomings in the consciousness of Americans.

Ice Cream: Swill or Swell?

Although a half cup of ice cream was considered somewhat more healthful than the nutrient description for the dessert, both were perceived as relatively unhealthful compared to all of the other foods that Oakes and Slotterback examined.[4] However, of the dozen high-fat foods that were examined ice cream was perceived as one of the most healthful. The average health rating for ice cream was just behind peanut butter, which was the most highly regarded high-fat food (and was once considered a health food itself[28]), and a hamburger, which came in second. The most salient characteristics of the nutrient description for ½ cup of vanilla ice cream were fat content (11 percent of the daily value) and cholesterol content (10 percent of the daily value). Additionally, absolutely no vitamin and mineral reached 10 percent of the daily value (calcium only reached 8 percent of the daily value).[4] What factors might perhaps explain ice cream's healthful reputation in relationship to other high-fat foods like potato chips? First, an examination of milk, the primary ingredient of the savory dessert, may be helpful.

America's early food reformers, even those that had some otherwise farfetched notions about healthy eating, believed that milk was indeed wholesome fare. Historical figures like Graham, Kellogg and even Horace Fletcher endorsed milk consumption as long as it was fresh, unpasteurized, and unadulterated (some unscrupulous dealers sometimes watered down the milk, and then added chalk, plaster of Paris, and molasses[29]). Additionally, in Fletcher's case it was imperative to chew milk thoroughly before swallowing (no joke).[30] One exception was consumption of swill milk, coming from scrawny city-stabled cattle fed distillery mash, which was not considered wholesome in nineteenth-century America.[31] The peddling of shabby, watered down, and adulterated milk was once referred to in the mid-nineteenth century as "milk murder." [32]

Although the dairy industry has never been shy about touting the value of milk, early twentieth-century nutritional scientists, at least of the mainstream variety, were largely in agreement with the industry. Many highly regarded nutritionists considered milk the most important food for humans. For example, chemist Henry Sherman, one of America's leading nutritionists of the 1930s, argued that diets which included milk would extend the human life span.[33] Chemist Elmer McCollum, from Johns Hopkins University, a most notable pioneer in nutrition research, stated in 1918 that milk "is the most satisfactory single article of food which is suitable for consumption by man." McCollum went on to praise milk as "truly the ideal food"[34] and due to milk's perceived capacity to promote health and prevent (or even reverse) disease processes McCollum classified milk a "protective food" along with leafy vegetables such as spinach.[35, 36] Ironically, the two characters in American history who are likely most responsible for the wholesome reputation of spinach are Elmer McCollum and perhaps even more importantly Popeye the sailor man.[37]

Although both total dairy product and beverage milk consumption have declined a great deal since the 1950s[38] (largely due to concerns about fat and cholesterol content[39]), in the 1970s milk products were still being lauded often with no reservations concerning fat content. For example, one Harvard professor remarked milk "provides more nutritive value per serving than any other naturally occurring food."[40] However, to most Americans nowadays the wholesomeness of milk products depends to a large extent on the fat content of the product. Dairy products perceived to be low in fat are praised, particularly by women, where those considered to have excessive fat are viewed much more negatively.[4, 5]

Just like today there were dissenting opinions among the experts regarding the value of milk products. For instance, a more minor issue involved the fact that some Americans of the early twentieth century believed that combining dairy products with certain other foods (e.g., fruit, oysters, or crabs) in the same meal promoted dyspepsia.[41, 42] Although concerns about the purity and sanitation of milk extend back to the beginning of American history, several accounts of undesirable ingredients in milk were described in the 1930s. Chemist Ira Garard described an incident occurring in the 1930s where he and his students discovered by accident that the college cafeteria milk was adulterated with formaldehyde.[43] Arthur Kallett and Fredick Schlink considered milk to be nothing short of an overly propagandized pestilence to all Americans. Writing in 1933, the two documented a variety of perceived health hazards caused by milk consumption. To Kallett and Schlink milk was blatantly filthy fare due to the fact that it was an excellent breeding ground for disease-causing germs.[44] Two years later Frederick Schlink penned his own scandalous expose on the hazards of eating in America. Schlink devoted an entire chapter to the denunciation of dairy products and those who endorsed (or in his words propagandized) such products, whom he referred to as "faddists." Schlink warned that dangerous metals like copper and lead and other toxins like arsenic were common contaminates in milk and ice cream (a legacy of processing kettles and piping and improperly pastured cows). Counter to the views of McCollum who considered milk to be "protective" and the most wholesome food that humans could consume, Schlink viewed milk as an unnecessary, unhealthful, and artificially vitamized fad food that was often toxic and indigestible to humans (particularly adults). Schlink suggested that milk drinking causes irreparable damage to the stomach, cataracts, bladder stones, and malnutrition.[45] Additionally, milk causes "coated tongue, bad breath, and a feeling as if the world had gone to ruin." [46] Children fed too much milk become pale, constipated, had restless sleep, wet the bed, and often resorted to eating dirt.[47] Probably the most notable modern day opponent of milk consumption is pediatrician Frank Oski who penned a popular milk-maligning volume several years ago entitled, *Don't Drink Your Milk! New Frightening Medical Facts about the World's Most Overrated Nutrient.* Oski has blamed milk consumption for a variety of childhood health problems (e.g., ear infections, constipation, asthma, and skin conditions).[48]

Ice cream has been referred to by food historians as a symbol of America.[49] The average American slurps between five and six gallons of the savory concoction annually, more than any other country.[50] Elmer McCollum thought very highly of the frozen concoction, in fact, he remarked "when not adulterated with cheap fillers it is to be classified as a protective food."[51] However, Frederick Schlink was not impressed with the popular dessert. He related that although ice cream is often considered a health food by many of us misinformed Americans, space did not permit him to expound on the health hazards that develop from eating the overrated and "oversweetened dessert" (in fact, he related that a future book would be devoted to the task). However, he did go on to convey that ice cream often contains "colon bacteria (an indication of the most dangerous, disease-breeding contamination by filth)." [52] Ice cream that had been melted then refrozen was said to be particularly unsafe. Finally, according to Schlink ice cream and other sweets corrupted our taste.

Throughout the nineteenth century ice cream consumption, at least outside the home (e.g., in ice cream saloons and parlors), became primarily a feminine pursuit.[53] According to historian Richard Hooker this trend may have begun in the late eighteenth century.[54] Meanwhile concerns of the potential perils of ice cream as being filthy and adulterated increased. Ice cream purchased from street vendors was considered most suspect. Sweet-food historian Wendy Woloson strongly suggested that a negative racial bias towards the Italians who often peddled the frozen concoction was partially responsible for this belief. [55] Parenthetically, there were concerns during the first half of the twentieth century that consumption of dairy products would sissify our soldiers. Thus, in World War I the Army recommended that soldiers not drink milk.[56] A similar sentiment was expressed by some military personnel concerning ice cream consumption during World War II.[49]

Even some food faddists chimed in to praise dairy food consumption. Paradoxically, there were those who advocated milk for losing weight and others who embraced milk drinking as a means for enhancing one's girth.[57] The bananas and skim milk diet developed by Dr. George Harrop of Johns Hopkins University was popular during the depression era.[58] Faddist Gaylord Hauser generally considered milk unhealthful but lauded skim milk, as well as brewer's yeast, wheat germ, yogurt, and blackstrap molasses as being life extending "wonder" foods.[59] However, other pseudo-nutritionists condemned milk consumption as unnatural and a cause of ailments ranging from colds to cancers.[60] Another example would be the popular yet quackish nutritionist Adelle Davis who warned Americans against pasteurized or homogenized milk consumption throughout the mid twentieth century.[61]

Ice cream was considered more healthful than most of the other high-fat foods examined by Oakes and Slotterback and considered more healthful than its nutrient description because it is often assumed to possess high levels of at least several vitamins and minerals (as well as protein). This belief may be a legacy of milk's (and to a lesser extent ice cream's) healthful reputation among mainstream nutritionists and health gurus of the nineteenth and twentieth centuries. Other than concerns about contamination, adulteration, and the effemination of soldiers, ice cream was considered a healthy food until recently.

A Potato by any Other Name

Many nutritional authorities as well as lay Americans consider the potato to be inferior to other vegetables in terms of vitamin and mineral content.[4, 5] Additionally, tubers have a reputation for contributing to plumpness. One food historian referred to the potato as a "marginally valuable nutritional source" consisting of carbohydrates mostly, a few grams of protein, and some vitamin C.[62] Other students of nutrition revealed that potatoes are mostly starch "but that they do contain small amounts of protein and are a fairly good source of vitamin C."[63] Additionally, there were the nutritional authorities quoted in chapters one and three from Harvard who recently related that other than calories the potato is nutritionally insignificant.[64] Even more recently (i.e., January 2003) those same Harvard nutritional authorities conveyed "being mainly starch, potatoes do not confer the benefits seen for other vegetables."[65] Finally, according to Oakes and Slotterback the name "potato" was considered the least healthful of all the fruits and vegetables examined. On the other hand, the nutrient description for the potato was judged to be the most healthful of all the fruits and vegetables examined.[4, 5] In contrast to these negative views of the humble potato, according to the primary nutrient table provided by Jean Pennington, [6] an ordinary grubby potato with skin has high concentrations (i.e., at least 10 percent of the recommended daily value) of no less than eleven different vitamins and minerals as well as nine percent of our recommended daily protein. The vitamin and mineral profile of the potato is as follows (expressed as percentage of the daily value): vitamin A 0 percent, vitamin C 43 percent, vitamin B-1 15 percent, vitamin B-2 4 percent, niacin 17 percent, vitamin B-6 35 percent, vitamin B-12 0 percent, folic acid 6 percent, pantothenic acid 11 percent, potassium 24 percent, calcium 2 percent, phosphorus 12 percent, magnesium 14 percent, iron 15 percent, zinc 4 percent, copper 31 percent, manganese 23 percent. Additionally, although potatoes have very little of the mineral selenium or vitamins D and E, depending on preparation a potato does have in excess of 10 percent of the daily value of vitamin K. A comparison of these figures with those from the much more highly regarded carrot is nothing short of amazing: carrots have high concentrations of only two vitamins and minerals (three if vitamin K is included which does barely reach 10 percent of the daily value in a single raw carrot) and almost no protein. Even a potato without its skin has very respectable amounts of vitamins and minerals (no less than seven different vitamins and minerals reach or surpass 10 percent of the recommended daily value). What accounts for the discrepancy between the potato's name and description ratings of healthfulness and why is the spud in disrepute compared to other vegetables?

The potato (a.k.a. tuber, papata, spud, Murphy, or mickey[66]) was originally a South American vegetable, which found its way to

England over 400 years ago. Early on, the Europeans considered the potato to be exotic and not acceptable for eating. To most Europeans the potato was primarily considered an ornamental plant at first: "Stylish gentleman wore potato flowers in their buttonholes." [67] Even when it became well established as food in parts of Europe several hundred years ago it was not preferred. Potatoes were considered poor mans' food and even among the lower class the potato was a priority food source often only in desperate times (i.e., famines).[9] Early American colonists who had a greater abundance of more prestigious foods available than did the Europeans opted to ignore the lowly potato. Colonial Americans considered potatoes to be nothing short of outright poison. Perhaps this view that tubers were toxic is due, in part, to the fact that the potato is a member of a family of plants called nightshade: some varieties of nightshade which are common in the United States are in fact fairly toxic. Alternatively, possibly ethnic biases have shaped our views of the spud, the ordinary potato had been strongly linked to a perceived undesirable and unsavory lot (the despised Irish).[9] In fact, the potato was actually often referred to in the United States as the Irish potato and regarded as a poor man's filler.[68] Although potatoes became a staple American food in the nineteenth century they were seldom mentioned in accounts of pre American-revolution fare. It took the adventurousness of one of our plucky forefathers, Thomas Jefferson (a man considered notorious in regards to the unusual plants that he cultivated) to begin growing the unpretentious spud. Thus, Jefferson fostered changes in our attitude toward the scrubby tuber. Even after Americans resigned themselves to eating potatoes, they took care in their preparation of the tuber, for it was thought that only boiling could rid potatoes of their toxins. Boiling potatoes made them safely edible for it allowed their harmful ingredients to be leached into the water. Warnings as recent as 1904 alerted Americans to discard the water used to boil potatoes: the chemicals therein were dangerous and had been known to poison pets.[9] By 1925 there were no longer concerns about potato toxicity, at least among mainstream nutritional authorities (however, there were rumors that potato skins might be toxic as recent as twenty-five years ago[69]). Although Elmer McCollum felt that Americans often relied on potatoes too much in their diets, he related that it is certainly safe (though not popular) to feed infants potato juice.[70] However, even at this time the potato was still undervalued compared to other foods. For example, it is noteworthy that in the 1930s the much less nutritious raw apple was considered in some circles to be a "highly protective food" (although not by McCollum) but in the same classification system the nutrient-rich potato was described as one of the "less protective foods." [71] Parenthetically, it is an interesting fact that the tomato and potato have much in common: both originated in South America, both are of the nightshade family and were considered toxic by our ancestors, and Thomas Jefferson is often given credit for being one of the first cultivators of both tomatoes and potatoes in the United States.[9]

These days Americans generally consider vegetables to be extremely wholesome and nutritious foods. However, many Americans do not readily associate the potato with being a vegetable at least not to the extent that we do the carrot, for example.[4] Although potatoes never were considered a prestigious food to most Americans, in many regions of the United States they became the most commonly consumed vegetable in the nineteenth century. In the early decades of the twentieth century, potatoes were recommended highly by our own federal government. Perhaps due to the fact that the potato was (and to a lesser extent still is) truly a staple component of the American diet it has become disassociated from other vegetables. Interestingly, one source produced by the federal government in 1918 covered the potato in much greater detail in the chapter devoted to cereals, rather than the passage depicting fruits and vegetables.[72] Similarly, potatoes are frequently considered separate from other vegetables in accounts of vegetable consumption. For example, American food historians often distinguish potatoes from other vegetables[73] and the United States Department of Agriculture (USDA) provides historical trends of potato consumption and an entirely separate category for all other vegetables combined.[38] Additionally, dietary recommendations of the 1930s and 40s from the USDA show that potatoes were mentioned by name and considered separate from other fruits and vegetables. In the 1930s Americans were advised by the Department of Agriculture to eat one serving of potatoes or sweet potatoes daily. Interestingly by the mid-1950s the emphasis on tuber consumption was no longer evident in USDA dietary guidelines, instead the importance of eating dark green/yellow vegetables was stressed.[74, 75] References implicating potato consumption as a contributor to obesity were becoming evident by this time. As early as 1925 Elmer McCollum indicated that potatoes should be eaten "sparingly" if your goal is to reduce body weight.[76] Thus, the fact that potatoes lack prestige and are devalued in terms of healthfulness may in part be due to the fact that they are not closely connected in the consciousness of Americans to the highly regarded class of foods the we call vegetables. Nutritional scientists from Harvard who penned a recent *Scientific American* article endorsing changes in the food pyramid are encouraging this perspective by advising readers to use potatoes "sparingly" but all other vegetables "in abundance." Additionally, these Harvard authorities had this to say "The inclusion of potatoes as a vegetable in the USDA pyramid has little justification..."[65]

As you might now expect, Frederick Schlink also had something to say about potatoes. Schlink related that "experiments by a competent physiologist" have shown that high protein diets (e.g., meat, eggs, and fish) containing minimal amounts of carbohydrates (e.g., "potatoes and sweet fruits") prevents colds.[77] The potato's association with fast food as well as French fries and potato chips (both being potato products perceived as excessively fatty, salty, and lacking in vitamins and minerals) may also foster a negative reputation of the humble potato. Interestingly, there is little if any evidence that food faddists ever emphasized the nutritious (but devalued) potato in their dietary schemes.

Clearly, purveyors of nutritional wisdom (both legitimate and quackish) have largely overlooked the nutritionally impressive spud. And the reason for this oversight is due to the fact that the potato carries an enduring but lowly legacy from our distant past (i.e., before the advent of vitamins). Additionally, although never demonstrated in research, the scrubby potato may not connote the desired characteristic "freshness" to the extent of other fruits and vegetables in the consciousness of Americans.

Hamburgers: From Gutter to Greatness

Although both the name "hamburger" and the nutrient description for a hamburger are not considered healthful by college students or more mature adults (no high fat food is judged to be wholesome), the hamburger was considered one of the more healthful of the high-fat foods examined by Oakes and Slotterback.[4, 5] For example, although the nutrient descriptions for the two are similar, the name "hamburger" was considered much more healthful than the name "Snickers bar." [4, 5]

Hamburger historian David Gerard Hogan described the hamburger as "undeniably America's favorite food" and our "most identifiable ethnic food."[78] Although likely a controversial viewpoint, Hogan has argued that the fast-food industry has in large part "improved the collective diet" of Americans and has contributed positively to our society and the entire world.[79] On the other hand, fast food industry critic Eric Schlosser depicts the brutality of the slaughter houses and generally paints a much more seamy picture of the beef and fast food industries as promoters of disease, crime, illegal immigration, and social hardship.[80]

Whether loved or loathed the hamburger was an American innovation. At some historical moment in American culinary history an adventurous food vendor (motivated perhaps by desperation more than visionariness) slapped slabs of bread above and beneath a Hamburg Steak patty (i.e., a ground beef patty) and the hamburger was born. We know that this momentous event occurred in the late nineteenth or early twentieth centuries but who exactly was responsible for the innovation is disputed.[81]

Throughout most of American history (until the 1970s), and in spite of concerns about meat contamination and adulteration, beef connoted prestige and was considered wholesome American fare. However, in the early years of the twentieth century, hamburger (as well as hotdogs) had an unsavory reputation. Turn-of-the-century Americans were suspicious of ground beef, believing that it was ground because it was of poor quality, spoiled, or otherwise unsafe to eat. For this reason hamburgers were thought to be poor mans' food or "fair food." They were served primarily at portable lunch carts near factories, at carnivals, and when the circus came to town. Rarely if ever were hamburgers offered in restaurants. Thus, the challenge for the creators of White Castle, America's first hamburger chain, was to quickly improve the unwholesome reputation of the lowly hamburger.[82]

White Castle founders responded to America's hamburger apprehension with some careful planning and innovations. First, whiteness, which connoted sanitation and purity, was emphasized in terms of the uniforms required by the employees, exterior and interior walls of the buildings, and even in the name of the establishment. Similarly, White Castle founders hoped that the term "castle" would signify permanence, strength, and respect. Second, the meat used for the White Castle burgers was of high grade. And, the grinding of the beef and grilling of the burgers occurred directly behind the counter so that potentially wary customers could monitor the process. Third, the establishments and employees were clean, tidy, and attractive to patrons. And finally, to convince Americans that hamburgers were healthful and indeed contained essential nutrients, White Castle founders demonstrated that a University of Minnesota graduate student could eat nothing but White Castle hamburgers for thirteen weeks and maintain good health.[82] Although according to White Castle historian David Hogan the hamburger quickly shifted from being a disreputable fad food to a staple of the middle class diet, some nutrition authorities were rather slow to accept the hamburger as wholesome American Fare. Arthur Kallet and Frederick Schlink alerted their readers to hamburger hazards in their 1933 book, *100, 000, 000 Guinea Pigs*,

> The hamburger habit is just about as safe as walking in an orchard while the arsenic spray is being applied, and about as safe as getting your meat out of a garbage can standing in the hot sun. For, beyond all doubt, the garbage can is where much of the chopped meat sold by butchers belongs... [83]

Further, Kallet and Schlink warned that the sodium sulphite used to restore the odor, color and appearance of freshness in already spoiled ground beef was "itself of the most severe of all digestive and kidney hazards."[84] Coauthor Frederick Schlink penned his own muckraking treatise two years later where he denigrated all processed foods except fresh meat (as long as it was not hamburger of course) as well as milk and many fruits and vegetables.[26]

Hamburgers were certainly not the only type of fare that aroused the suspicions of Americans during this time period. The memories of the food atrocities depicted in *The Jungle* and related articles as well as concerns about food purity were still in the public consciousness. Any processed food, particularly if it was packaged (which prevented customers from seeing, smelling, and tasting the goods), generated fear.[85] To allay fears many food companies offered factory tours so that people could witness food processing methods and the conditions under which food was processed and packaged. Also, many food companies established a whimsical tradition in their ad campaigns by using elfin, cherubic, clownish, or Kewpie doll characters to promote their products and alleviate anxieties about their processed fare. Familiar examples would be the Campbell's Kids, Rice Krispies (Snap, Crackle, and Pop), and the Pillsbury doughboy. [85]

Concerns about meat adulteration arose again three or four decades back when, for example, Ralph Nader referred to the American staple as the "shamburger." [86] Further, the hamburger's very association with the fast-food industry and the much publicized outbreaks of E-coli which have been linked to the industry have likely contributed to the burger's downfall in prestige in the consciousness of Americans.[80] However, there is little doubt that the most formidable assault against the hamburger began in the 1970s (Americans beef consumption had been increasing until this time[38]) with the campaign against dietary fat.

A food's level of dietary fat has been shown to be the most influential determinant of a food's reputations.[3, 4, 5] It is reasonable to assume that the campaign against dietary fat has likely elicited huge shifts in the American public's perception of hamburger healthfulness. Perhaps, the fact that hamburgers are judged to be healthful in comparison to other high-fat foods, reflects the positive view of the burger before the assault on dietary fat. It might also be argued that the fast-food enterprise, which figuratively pulled the slimy and disreputable hamburger out of the garbage in the early decades of the twentieth century, may also have ultimately besmeared the burger's health reputation in the last half of the century.

Summary and Conclusions

On the one hand it is fairly obvious that dramatic shifts in the public's perception of foods can occur as a result of consistent bombardment of specific nutritional messages (e.g., natural is good and dietary fat is bad). On the other hand, it appears that the modern reputations of many foods are influenced by food beliefs and attitudes from our distant past (before the advent of vitamins). Clearly, the apple's rich history in America has blurred its nutritional shortcomings in the eyes of many of those who disseminate nutritional information. These legacies concerning a food's status are not only enduring but are also held sacred by many Americans including those who are considered knowledgeable about food healthfulness. It is not politically correct to challenge the status (in terms of healthfulness) of the mighty apple. Some may view such information as un-American or some sort nutritional blasphemy. However, at the risk of sounding glib, this line of research strongly suggests that we have many "protected beliefs" concerning food nutrition and healthfulness.

Notes

1. M. Cussler and M. L. de Give, *Twixt the cup and the lip* (New York: Twayne Publishers 1952), 152.
2. J. W. Bennett, Food and social status in a rural society, *American Sociological Review* 8 (1943), 561-569.
3. M. E. Oakes, Differences in Judgments of Food Healthfulness by Young and Elderly Women, *Food Quality and Preference* in press.
4. M. E. Oakes and C. S. Slotterback, What's in a name? A comparison of men's and women's judgements about food names and their nutrient contents, *Appetite* 36 (2001[b]), 29-40.
5. M. E. Oakes and C. S. Slotterback, Judgements of food healthfulness: food name stereotypes in adults over age 25, *Appetite* 37 (2001[c]), 1-8.
6. J. A. T. Pennington, *Bowes and Church's Food values of portions commonly used* (Philadelphia, PA: Lippincott 1998).
7. T. Hensley, Apples of your eye, *Smithsonian* (Nov. 2002), 111-118.
8. No author, Johnny Appleseed. A pioneer hero. *Harper's New Monthly Magazine* XLIII (Nov. 1871), 830-836.
9. W. Root and R. de Rochemont, *Eating in America: a history* (New York: William Morrow and Company, Inc. 1976), 233.
10. G. Titelman, *Random house dictionary of American's popular proverbs and sayings* 2nd edition (New York: Random House 2000).
11. H. L. Mencken, *A new dictionary of quotations on historical principles from ancient and modern sources* (New York: Alfred A. Knoff 1962).
12. *The Ladies' Home Magazine*, 16 (Dec. 1860), 372.
13. cited in M. Stacey, Consumed: *Why Americans love, hate, and fear food* (New York: Simon and Schuster 1994), 115-116.
14. C. C. Furnas and S. M. Furnas, *Man, Bread and destiny*, (New York: Reynal and Hitchcock 1937).
15. E. V. McCollum, *A history of nutrition: the sequence of ideas in nutrition investigations* (Boston: Houghton Mifflin Company 1957), 168.
16. R. O. Cummings, *The American and his food* (New York: Arno Press and The New York Times 1970), 257.
17. V. Herbert and S. Barrett, *Vitamins and "health" foods: The great American hustle* (Philadelphia: George F. Stickley Company 1981), 89.
18. W. M. Johnson, The rise and fall of food fads, *The American Mercury* 28 (1933), 475-478.
19. F. J. Stare and E. M. Whelan, *Eat ok—feel ok!: Food facts and your health* (North Quincy, MA: The Christopher Publishing House 1978), 230.
20. E. V. McCollum and N. Simmonds, *Food, nutrition and health* (Baltimore: published by the authors 1925), 60.
21. Cummings, *The American and his food*, 43-44.
22. A. Kallet and F. J. Schlink, *100, 000, 000 guinea pigs* (New York: Grosset and Dunlap 1933), 47-60.

23. F. J. Schlink, *Eat drink and be wary* (New York: Covici Friede Publishers 1935), 42.
24. Schlink, *Eat drink and be wary*, 64.
25. Schlink, *Eat drink and be wary*, 42.
26. Schlink, *Eat drink and be wary*.
27. Kallet and Schlink, *100, 000, 000 guinea pigs*, 25-29.
28. R. M. Deutsch, *The nuts among the berries* (New York: Ballantine Books 1967), 133.
29. Cummings, *The American and his food*, 55.
30. R. M. Deutsch, *The nuts among the berries* (New York: Ballantine Books 1967) 72 and 120.
31. Cummings, *The American and his food*, 53.
32. R. J. Hooker, *Food and drink in America a history* (New York: The Bobbs-Merrill Company, Inc. 1981), 129.
33. H. Levenstein, *Paradox of plenty: A social history of eating in modern America* (New York: Oxford University Press 1993), 14.
34. E. V. McCollum, *The newer knowledge of nutrition: The use of food for the preservation of vitality and health* (New York: The Macmillan Company 1923), 150.
35. McCollum, *The newer knowledge of nutrition*, 343.
36. McCollum and Simmonds, *Food, nutrition and health*, 43.
37. Cummings, *The American and his food*, 152.
38. USDA, *Agriculture Fact Book* 2000.
39. Hooker, *Food and drink in America: A history*, 340-341.
40. Stare and Whelan, *Eat ok – feel ok: Food facts and your health*, 21
41. McCollum and Simmonds, *Food, nutrition and health*, 81.
42. Johnson, The rise and fall of food fads, *The American Mercury*.
43. I. D. Garard, *The story of food* (Westport, Connecticut: The AVI Publishing Company, Inc. 1974), 69-70.
44. Kallet and Schlink, *100, 000, 000 guinea pigs*.
45. Schlink, *Eat drink and be wary*.
46. Schlink, *Eat drink and be wary*, 232.
47. Schlink, *Eat drink and be wary*, 233.
48. F. A. Oski, *Don't drink your milk! New frightening medical facts about the world's most overrated nutrient* (Syracuse, NY: Mollica 1983).
49. Root and de Rochemont, *Eating in America: a history*, 423.
50. W. S. Arbuckle, *Ice cream* (The AVI Publishing Company, Inc. 1972), 10.
51. McCollum and Simmonds, *Food, nutrition and health*, 68.
52. Schlink, *Eat drink and be wary*, 248.
53. W. A. Woloson, *Refined tastes: Sugar, confectionery, and consumers in nineteenth-century America* (Baltimore: The Johns Hopkins University Press 2002), 105.
54. Hooker, *Food and drink in America: A history*, 79.
55. Woloson, *Refined tastes,* 105.
56. Federal Security Agency, Office of the Director of Defense, Health and Welfare Services. *Proceedings of the national nutrition conference for defense* (May 1941), 25.
57. H. Schwartz, *Never satisfied: A cultural history of diets, fantasies and fat* (New York: The Free Press 1986).
58. Levenstein, *Paradox of plenty,* 14.
59. J. V. Young, *The medical messiahs: A social history of health quackery in twentieth-century America* (Princeton, New Jersey: Princeton University Press 1967), 340.

60. Stare and Whelan, *Eat ok—feel ok!: Food facts and your health*, 19
61. Stare and Whelan, *Eat ok—feel ok!: Food facts and your health*, 229
62. R. A. Sokolov, *Why we eat what we eat* (New York: Summit Books 1991), 125.
63. Stare and Whelan, *Eat ok—feel ok!: Food facts and your health*, 100.
64. CNN.com - Elizabeth Cohen: The Skinny on 'good fats'—July 8, 2002: Http// www.cnn.com/2002/HE...fitness/07/08/cohen.fat.otsc/index.ht
65. W. C. Willett, M. J. Stampfer, Rebuilding the food pyramid, *Scientific American* (January 2003), 64-71.
66. M. E. Lowenberg, E.N. Todhunter, E. D. Wilson, J. R. Savage, J. L. Lubawski, *Food and Man* 2nd edition (New York: John Wiley and Sons 1974), 99.
67. B. Norman, *Tales of the table: A history of Western cuisine* (Englewood Cliffs, NJ: Prentice-Hall, Inc 1972), 264.
68. Hooker, *Food and drink in America: A history*, 231.
69. R. W. Lacey, *Hard to swallow: A brief history of food* (Cambridge University Press 1994)
70. McCollum and Simmonds, *Food, nutrition and health*, 17.
71. Cummings, *The American and his food*, 257.
72. U. S. Food Administration, *Food saving and sharing* (New York: Doubleday, Page and Company 1918).
73. C. Van Syckle, Some pictures of food consumption in the United States: part 1. 1630-1860. *Journal of the American Dietetic Association* 19 (1945), 511.
74. C. Davis and E. Saltos, Dietary Recommendations and how they have changed over time. In *America's eating habits: Changes and consequences.* US Department of Agriculture, Economic Research Service, Food and Rural Economic Division, Agriculture Information Bulletin No. 750.
75. New wartime nutrition chart, *Medicine and the War* 122 (1943) 607-608.
76. McCollum and Simmonds, *Food, nutrition and health*, 100.
77. Schlink, *Eat drink and be wary*, 309.
78. D. G. Hogan, *Selling 'em by the sack* (New York: New York University Press 1999), 175.
79. Hogan, *Selling 'em by the sack*, 177-178.
80. E. Schlosser, *Fast food nation: The dark side of the all-American meal* (New York: Houghton Mifflin Company 2001).
81. J. Tennyson, *Hamburger heaven* (New York: Hyperion 1993).
82. Hogan, *Selling 'em by the sack.*
83. Kallet and Schlink, *100, 000, 000 guinea pigs*, 38.
84. Kallet and Schlink, *100, 000, 000 guinea pigs*, 39.
85. S. Strasser, *Satisfaction guaranteed: The making of the American mass market* (Washington: Smithsonian Institutional Press 1989).
86. Levenstein, *Paradox of plenty*, 171.

Conclusion

The idea that nutrition beliefs are all too often not in agreement with nutritional facts or established science is a constant theme throughout this volume. Attempts have been made to provide the reader with information pertaining to how these beliefs have become engrained into the American consciousness. Perhaps more than ever before in American history the time appears to be right for a volume that explores these sacred beliefs. Americans more than ever are being bombarded with the message that we should avoid some of the foods that we appreciate most (e.g., the hamburger and chocolate). Further, more and more people are convinced that an extreme adjustment in the type of foods that are available to us is necessary. For example, for better or worse legal arguments are currently being marshaled with the hopes of limiting the availability of our "bad foods." Although the work presented in this volume is unique in its exploration of nutritional beliefs and the science in support of those beliefs others have taken a more emotional tone. For example, one author recently conveyed the following, "Many of the choices people make in an effort to improve their nutritional well-being are based on sweeping generalities, half-baked data, ignorance, prejudice, and superstition."[1]

Further, others have provided insight into the potential motives behind dietary changes and to some degree challenged our modern views of eating for health. For instance, Michelle Stacey described a few years back what she called a "peculiarly American assumption" that by eating "good" foods and avoiding the "bad" ones we can "control our own mortality—that we can put off our own deaths, with the ultimate unspoken hope that we might outsmart death entirely." According to Stacey, the basic idea (that by eating reputable foods we can control our health and mortality) is relatively new in American history and was first popularized by William Sylvester Graham. Stacey also emphasized the importance of our faith in science and technology "as forces that will eventually change all the rules in our favor."[2]

At times throughout this volume attempts have been made to describe what some might suggest are the fallibilities of the science that we trust so much (e.g., the squabbles within the scientific community over the health value of decreasing salt and fat intake). Others have also suggested that scientific data often is susceptible to misinterpretation based on the preconceived beliefs of the investigator that can be overly influenced by the current prevailing views in science and society. Physician Alvan Feinstein provided an example depicting how the pathogenesis of pellagra (which we now know is due to niacin deficiency) was at first thought to be infectious and perhaps inherited. This was because reliable scientific data showing that the disease was often more common among certain families and neighborhoods was interpreted to fit with the prevailing scientific views of that era.[3] The argument could be made that the social/scientific pendulum is now positioned differently so that modern day health problems, ailments, discomforts, and worries are too often attributed to eating the "wrong" foods. For example, it would not be uncommon these days for someone who is overweight or at least perceives him or herself to be overweight to be given advice to change the type of foods consumed or even take certain vitamins, supplements, or herbal remedies. If so, such advice would likely be stated with certainty and authority. For instance, the following was quoted from the jacket of a newly published diet/nutrition book. "This is a book that will let you live longer, reduce your need for medications, and improve you health dramatically. It is a book that will change the way you want to eat. But most important of all, if you follow the *Eat to Live* diet, you will lose weight faster than you ever thought possible."[4] Although these sorts of books are abundant and always herald categorical answers to difficult questions, the truth is researchers are somewhat perplexed by Americans' weight problems. One authority from the Centers for Disease Control and Prevention offered the following a few years back, "we have not clearly identified the major changes in eating behavior or activity sufficient to account for the recent rapid increase in obesity."[5] Some investigators have attributed a portion of the increase in numbers of overweight adults to smoking cessation. Astonishingly, others have at least suggested that perhaps Americans are not getting fatter but just heavier. These folks are putting a positive spin on Americans' weight problems by suggesting that increased body weight may be attributed to increases in lean-body mass due to exercise rather than to body fat. As the reader might expect, few experts are endorsing this perspective.[5]

Perhaps the safest and least controversial explanations for America's escalating rates of obesity involve increased physical inactivity and just plain overeating. Increased portion sizes of foods sold both in grocery stores and in restaurants may in part explain why Americans are more portly than ever.[6] Dietician Lisa Drayer recently conveyed due to the popularity of eating out "we're getting a distorted view of what portion sizes are. We're not likely to make a distinction between restaurant sizes and real sizes when going home."[7] Some of the greatest increases in portions have been observed for Mexican dishes, salty snack foods, hamburgers and soft drinks.[6] Nutritionist Marion Nestle has found that if we eat the average American muffin (about six ounces) we get triple of what the USDA indicates is appropriate for a serving of muffin (two ounces).[8] Further, Paul Rozin discovered that even the fruits and vegetables sold in stores in the United States are much larger than those sold in Europe.[9] In fact, increased portion sizes together with more physical inactivity likely go a long way in explaining America's ever increasing tendency toward plumpness. Astonishingly, one source indicated that the average American burns 800 fewer calories per day compared to just two decades ago.[10] Certainly, some nutritional authorities would likely dispute the magnitude of this reported change in activity level.

At least a few Americans have expressed the belief (and some food researchers would agree) that we are bombarded these days with scientific information about healthy eating. No doubt, thanks to innovations like the computer there is more scientific information available to us than ever before (e.g., increased numbers of journals published). Further, statistical procedures that several decades ago would have taken the average scientist hours or even days now can be completed in minutes or seconds. Given the fact that statistical procedures take such little time, the appropriate sequence of steps in the scientific method often become altered. That is, hypotheses are more often determined after data analyses rather than before. Thus, the data dredging and retroactive changes in hypotheses in which certain salt researchers have been accused (discussed in chapter four) are more common than ever. It is easy for researchers to complete one complex statistical analysis after another until results are found that conform with their existing beliefs. Hypotheses are then developed that fit with the sought after results and the investigator's belief system or politics.[3] The research findings are likely further filtered through the popular media. Thus, it might be argued that Americans end up assimilating somewhat biased information about eating and health in general, and some are put off by the apparent contradictions

It has occurred to some critics that certain types of scientific exploration are particularly suspect. A few years ago Gary Taubes reported in *Science* magazine the problems of epidemiological research that attempts to uncover associations between environmental agents (e.g., dietary fat) and disease (e.g., cancer). Such studies have been said to promote an "epidemic of anxiety"[11] and according to the epidemiologists themselves "are so plagued with biases, uncertainties, and methodological weakness that they may be inherently incapable of accurately discerning such weak associations."[11] As one epidemiologist put it when referring to potential environmental hazards, "what's very hard to do is to tell a little thing from nothing at all." Another admitted, "we are fast becoming a nuisance to society" and that "we may unintentionally do more harm than good."[11] The solution offered by the scientists was that "the press must become more skeptical." As things stand now results from medical journals are "misconstrued by the lay press to be more definite than they really are"[11] and that the number of "false alarms" disseminated by the press are nothing short of alarming. However, health reporters become rankled with such comments and tend to blame the scientific journals for touting weak studies that over-dramatize potential health hazards and are not in agreement with the bulk of the research on the subject.[11]

These potential problems with the abundance and dissemination of scientific information along with historical legacies that persist for many foods as well as food industry propaganda likely explain to a large degree why certain foods reputations often do not correspond with nutrient contents. Perhaps no prudent and knowledgeable person has actually commented that dietary fat is the single most important nutrient to monitor in order to ensure health and longevity but one would certainly think so from attending to media coverage on nutrition. As stated in a previous chapter, the best that can be hoped is that this writing will foster a healthy skepticism about the abundance of messages (even those with a mainstream perspective) concerning diet and nutrition that we encounter routinely in our lives and to get more people talking about this issue. Many of the statements provided in this volume suggesting that food beliefs are often not in agreement with nutritional facts can easily be verified by the reader. The reader is encouraged to compare the vitamin and mineral content of reputable foods (e.g., apples and carrots) and those that are less reputable or infamous (e.g., potatoes and Big Macs).

Notes

1. M. Stacey, *Consumed: Why Americans love, hate, and fear food* (New York: Simon and Schuster 1994), 18.
2. M. Stacey, *Consumed:* 22-23.
3. A. R. Feinstein, Fraud, distortion, delusion, and consensus: The problems of human and natural deception in epidemiologic science, *The American Journal of Medicine* 84 (1988) 475-478.
4. J. Fuhrman, *Eat to live: The revolutionary formula for fast and sustained weight loss* (New York, NY: Little, Brown, and Company 2003).
5. G. Taubes, As obesity rates rise, experts struggle to explain why, *Science* 280 (1998) 1367-1368.
6. S. J. Nielsen and B. M. Popkin, Patterns and trends in food portion sizes 1977-1198, *Journal of the American Medical Association* 289 (2003) 450-453.
7. A. Fox, Study: Americans super-sizing at home, too, CNN.com January 23, 2003
8. B. Liebman, The pressure to eat, *Nutrition Action Newsletter* July/August (1998).
9. P. Rozin, *Learning about everything from studying food.* Paper presented at the 16th annual University of Scranton Psychology Conference, Scranton, PA (February, 2001).
10. K. Griffin, Rebel against a sedentary life, *Health* April (1997) 83-87.
11. G. Taubes, Epidemiology faces its limits, *Science* 269 (1995) 164-169.

Index

Hitler, 34
Hogan, David Gerard, 128, 129
Honey, 21, 94, 97
Hooker, Richard, 122
Hotdogs, 13-14, 37, 68, 69, 128
Human flesh consumption, 31
Hypertension (see blood pressure), 71
    and race, 83-84, 85
    and salt intake, 72, 73, 77, 82, 84, 85
    protein intoxication theory, 72-73
    rodent model for, 75
    theories concerning salt, 82-84
Hypoglycemia, 102, 106-107
Hyponatremia (water intoxication), 70

Ice cream (see craving), 92, 104
    and femininity, 98, 122, 123
    consumption in America, 122
    nutrient profile, 120
    reputation of, 119-120
    warnings against, 122-123
Improving Your Child's Behavior Chemistry, 102
Indigestion (dyspepsia), 25, 28, 50, 72, 118, 121
    on death certificates, 53
International Lists of Diseases and Causes of Death, 53
Intersalt study, 75, 84-85

Jackson, James A., 27
Jefferson, Thomas, 96, 125
Jungle, The, 32, 129
Junk food, 5, 8, 13
    taxation of, 13, 58

Kallet, Arthur, 119, 121, 129
Kellogg, John Harvey, 27-28, 120
Kempner, Wallace: and his diet, 73-74
Kentucky Fried Chicken (KFC), 18
Keys, Ancel, 53-54, 100

Lappe, Frances, 29
Levenstein, Harvey, 34
Lipoproteins (LDL, HDL), 46, 60, 62
Liquor, 47
Lithium (see salt substitution)
Livestock hormones, 35, 37
Low fat
    diets, 50, 56, 61, 62, 76
    foods, 4-5, 10, 57

Mad Cow Disease, 38-39
Margarine, 14-15, 29
Masturbation, 26, 99
Mayo Clinic, 34
Mayonnaise, 49
McCollum, Elmer, 118, 120, 121, 122, 125-126, 127
McDonald's, 51
McGovern, George, 54, 75
Meat (see hamburger), 54, 55
    and disease, 28, 31, 38-39
    eating and sex and aggression, 25, 26, 28, 30, 50
Inspection Law, 32
Pork, 50-51
    symbol of prosperity, 29
Mercury, 13, 35
Milk, 14, 54, 55, 105
    as protective food, 120, 122
    fads, 123
    origins of reputation, 120-122
    warnings against, 121-122, 123
Multiple sclerosis, 45

Nader, Ralph, 37, 130
Name versus description research, 5-12, Figures 1.1, 1.2, Table 1.1
National Institute of Health, 55
Natural
    on food labels, 18-19, 35-36
    origin of importance in America, 26
Nestle, Marion, 18, 137
New York Times Magazine, 61
Novocain, 69
Nutritional Epidemiology, 46
Nutritional science potential problems, 59, 136, 137-138
Nuts (see fat), 48, 51-52
Nutrition Labeling and Education Act (NLEA), 20, 40

Oakes, Mike, 3-4, 9, 59, 119, 123, 124, 127
Oat bran products, 29
Obesity (see sugar, fat)
    portion sizes and inactivity, 136-137
Olestra (see fat substitutes), 56-57
Olive oil, 48, 51
100,000,000 Guinea Pigs, 129
Organic
    as more nutritious, 19-20